DATE DUE

AUG 2 3 2011			

GAYLORD   PRINTED IN U.S.A.

It Happened to Me

Series Editor: Arlene Hirschfelder

Books in the It Happened to Me series are designed for inquisitive teens digging for answers about certain illnesses, social issues, or lifestyle interests. Whether you are deep into your teen years or just entering them, these books are gold mines of up-to-date information, riveting teen views, and great visuals to help you figure out stuff. Besides special boxes highlighting singular facts, each book is enhanced with the latest reading list, websites, and an index. Perfect for browsing, there's loads of expert information by acclaimed writers to help parents, guardians, and librarians understand teen illness, tough situations, and lifestyle choices.

1. *Learning Disabilities: The Ultimate Teen Guide,* by Penny Hutchins Paquette and Cheryl Gerson Tuttle, 2003.
2. *Epilepsy: The Ultimate Teen Guide,* by Kathlyn Gay and Sean McGarrahan, 2002.
3. *Stress Relief: The Ultimate Teen Guide,* by Mark Powell, 2002.
4. *Making Sexual Decisions: The Ultimate Teen Guide,* by L. Kris Gowen, Ph.D., 2003.
5. *Asthma: The Ultimate Teen Guide,* by Penny Hutchins Paquette, 2003.
6. *Cultural Diversity: Conflicts and Challenges: The Ultimate Teen Guide,* by Kathlyn Gay, 2003.
7. *Diabetes: The Ultimate Teen Guide,* by Katherine J. Moran, 2004.
8. *When Will I Stop Hurting? Teens, Loss, and Grief: The Ultimate Teen Guide,* by Edward Myers, 2004.
9. *Volunteering: The Ultimate Teen Guide,* by Kathlyn Gay, 2004.
10. *Organ Transplant: A Survival Guide for Recipients and Their Families: The Ultimate Teen Guide,* by Tina P. Schwartz, 2005.
11. *Medications: The Ultimate Teen Guide,* by Cheryl Gerson Tuttle, 2005.
12. *Image and Identity: Becoming the Person You Are,* by L. Kris Gowen, Ph.D., Ed.M., and Molly C. McKenna, Ph.D., 2005.
13. *Apprenticeship,* by Penny Hutchins Paquette, 2005.
14. *Cystic Fibrosis: The Ultimate Teen Guide,* by Melanie Ann Apel, 2006.

Cystic Fibrosis

The Ultimate Teen Guide

Melanie Ann Apel

It Happened to Me, No. 14

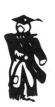

The Scarecrow Press, Inc.
Lanham, Maryland • Toronto • Oxford
2006

SCARECROW PRESS, INC.

Published in the United States of America
by Scarecrow Press, Inc.
A wholly owned subsidiary of
The Rowman & Littlefield Publishing Group, Inc.
4501 Forbes Boulevard, Suite 200, Lanham, Maryland 20706
www.scarecrowpress.com

PO Box 317
Oxford
OX2 9RU, UK

British Library Cataloguing in Publication Information Available

Library of Congress Cataloging-in-Publication Data

Apel, Melanie Ann.
  Cystic fibrosis : the ultimate teen guide / Melanie Ann Apel.
    p. cm. — (It happened to me ; no. 14)
  Includes bibliographical references and index.
  ISBN-13: 978-0-8108-4821-4 (hardcover : alk. paper)
  ISBN-10: 0-8108-4821-X (hardcover : alk. paper)
  1. Cystic fibrosis. 2. Cystic fibrosis in children. I. Title. II. Series.
RC858.C95A74 2006
618.92'372—dc22

                                                    2005022073

This book is dedicated with love to my dear friends Katie Kocelko and Chad Lucci. You are my inspirations!

I also dedicate this book to Anika and Mackenzie Bradley, who bring much joy into my life and the lives of my little boys. Anika, may you have a long and healthy life so that you may indeed marry Hayden some day!

This book is written in memory of my friends Troy Morrison, Angela Dibbern, Cristina Shadle, Jimmy Curry, Jenny DiBiase, Mike DiBiase, Amy Thom, Jessica Denny, and George Paulosky. You left the greatest marks on my life; you are still part of me.

And in memory of the friends I made at cystic fibrosis camp who taught me so much: Angela Budnieski, Brandy Miller, Fonda Rae Langston, Kelly Hutchings, Lisa Zepeda, Marc Guisinger, Nicole Guisinger, Mikey Thurson, Kimberlee Pilarczyk, Steve McMahon, Jennifer Cherry, Walter Johnson, Christina Schreiber, Christy Anderson, Cassondra Ditzler, Elyce MacCarthy, Jeremy Becker, Arnold Hoyer, Brian Conklin, Chris Gubelman, David Bailey, David Sellers, Douglas Caliendo, Evelyn Shavers, Jeff (whose last name I don't recall but who looked like Troy), John Ozga, José Burke, Kelly Kovach, Nicolette Vach, Shane Carter, Tangela Swan, Tasha Patton, and finally, courageously, Mike Williams.

In addition, this book is in memory of those I cared for at Children's Memorial Hospital: Lisa Cochran, Kathrin Lundquist, little Jessica Formhals, Christopher Downey, Shekeitheia Gordon, Bob Fisher, Sharita Kelly, Kristine Murphy, Thais VonDahlen, Julia Nicole Krasny, Natalie Elizabeth Lukoff, Sharon Talbert, Devon Davis, and Children's Memorial nurse Rosa DiFranco.

And most especially, this book is in memory of Alex Deford, who changed my whole life by bringing me here in the first place.

With all my love . . .

And now after all these years, your voices will be heard, and you will tell the others, "You are not alone."

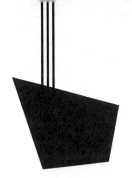

Contents

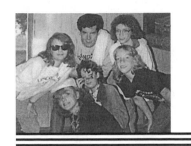

Contents

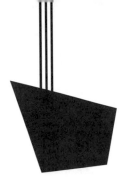

Medical Disclaimer

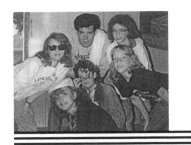

While the information presented within is factual, it is not intended for purposes of self-diagnosis or self-medication. If you suspect a case of cystic fibrosis or if you have cystic fibrosis and wish to change or try new treatments, consult with your physician. The stories you will read reflect the experiences and opinions of those telling them. Only the names of those represented in this book who wished anonymity have been changed. These names are indicated by an asterisk (*). All others are the real names of people who were gracious enough to share their stories for the purpose of this book.

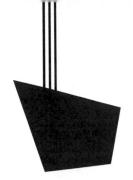

Acknowledgments

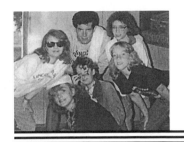

I wish to thank my family for allowing cystic fibrosis (CF) to touch their lives as it has touched mine, even though they didn't have to. Thank you to my sister, Mindy S. Apel, for timely and accurate research assistance, artistic talent, and love and support not only for this project but also for my involvement with CF over the course of nineteen years. Thank you Hayden and Alec Bonnell for being born healthy and for napping so Mommy could work. Thank you to my parents Carol and Darwin Apel: Mom, for having the courage to drop me off at CF camp so many years ago, for typing so willingly, and for babysitting with Dad when Hayden and Alec wouldn't nap, as well as for your unconditional love and support in general and specifically in terms of my CF dedication. Thank you to Michael Bonnell, for finding your way to Children's Memorial Hospital, too, and for all the little things and the big things, and especially for the crazy red head and the blue-eyed baby.

Thank you to my friends, Michele Hammer Ottenfeld for willingness to type; Cathy Carnevale for letting me bounce things off her; Chad Lucci who answered questions, read, typed, approved, and encouraged me when I just wasn't so sure I was doing a good job with this book; and Tina P. Schwartz for her insight, support, encouragement, and most especially for the lead that allowed me to *finally* write a book about cystic fibrosis. I wish to thank respiratory therapists Joanne Salazar and Cathy O'Malley for their CF expertise in approving the medical information in this book. Thank you to Brent Wineinger, for the essential photoshopping, and to Melody White, for providing last-minutes stats. I also wish to extend unparalleled gratitude to the

Acknowledgments

cleanup typists, Carol Apel, Mindy Apel, Chad Lucci, and Leah K., without whom the lost pages would never have been recovered and all would have been permanently gone; I could never have accomplished this without you. I owe you one!

Thank you to all my other wonderful friends, old and new—too many to name—who agreed to be interviewed for this book, even when it meant sharing very intimate and sometimes painful details of your lives. Thank you to the parents of Angela Budnieski, Angela Dibbern, Brandy Miller, Cassie Ditzler, Cris Shadle, Jenny DiBiase, Troy Morrison, Kimberlee Pilarczyk, and Lisa Zepeda for granting me permission to use their children's words and photos throughout this book to preserve their precious memories on paper forever. Speaking with each of you after all these years brought back so many beautiful memories, while also reminding me how important my work here really is. I really miss your kids! Thank you to Ken DiBiase, Kerry and Maggie Sheehan, Margaret Thom, and Katie Kocelko, who shared their stories with such honesty all those years ago and who have waited with such patience for this book! And though they are no longer with us, I wish to extend posthumous thanks to Mike DiBiase, Kimberlee Pilarczyk, and Jennifer Cherry, who let me interview them so long ago, letting me take a personal glimpse into the struggles they lived through with such dignity every day. And to Amy Thom, whose amazing and miraculous story launched my writing career; I owe you so much, Amy! And I'm so sorry you aren't here to see this book you helped create.

Thank you to the amazing people on the Cystic-L Listserve—again, too many to name, but you know who you are—who always came through for me with answers to my *never-ending* questions. There are many others who added tidbits here or there, filled in gaps, or provided some fact— thank you for helping me complete this project. I also wish to thank the entire CF "community"—those whom I have known and lost and those still fighting their battle—for taking me in and accepting me as one of your own, for making me an "honorary cystic," and for showing me what it means to be strong, brave, and full of life!

And, finally, thank you to Frank Deford for bringing Alex into my life.

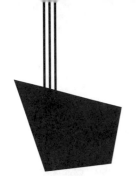

Introduction

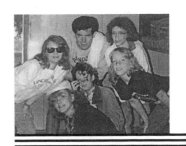

July 4, 1986. In a northern suburb of Chicago, Illinois, the sun begins to shine through clouds, eagerly eliminating all traces of the early morning's rainfall. A nervously excited 18-year-old girl and her mother drive up through the gates of a shabby old overnight camp. Thus begins the story of a girl and an adventure that would take a lifetime to unfold.

It all began in the spring of 1986 when the girl read a book written by Frank Deford about his daughter, Alexandra. The book, *Alex: The Life of a Child*, and the television movie of the same name, which aired that spring, told the poignant, true story of a little girl who had an incurable disease called cystic fibrosis. Author Frank Deford described his daughter's brief and beautiful time on earth before cystic fibrosis brought her eight-year life to a close.

"I was deeply moved by this story," the girl says. The story touched the girl more than anything had before, and she felt a profound and inexplicable need to become involved, to help, to maybe even make a difference. And truthfully, "I had to 'meet' Alex," the girl says, "and I knew the only way to do that was to know other kids like her. She was such an amazing little spirit; she touched me so much through her father's words. I had to bring this amazing presence into my life." Except she couldn't meet Alex because Alex had already been gone for several years. But what if the girl could meet other children like Alex? Maybe they could help her understand this beautiful little girl and the brave battle she fought against a cruel and unrelenting disease.

The girl looked up cystic fibrosis in the yellow pages. She called the Cystic Fibrosis Foundation and made an inquiry as to possible summer volunteer opportunities. She was offered two options: helping with a bike-a-thon or attending a weeklong overnight camp. Would she be brave enough to set aside her lifelong reluctance to be away from her family and specifically her fear of going away to summer camp?

"I never actually thought to myself, 'I can't do this,'" the girl says now. "Something about this opportunity was different from anything else I'd ever considered. I felt compelled. I had to go. It was so joyously unlike me! I grilled the camp director for all sorts of details, and she did her best to set my mind at ease. I was afraid, but once I had made up my mind to go, there was no turning back." The girl hoped one of her friends might join her on this adventure, but all of her friends refused. "I don't think I could spend a week with sick kids, watching them all dying," one friend told her.

So, the girl packed summer clothes ("Don't bring too many clothes," her father advised), a sleeping bag, snacks, a camera, and a journal. Then, rather than attending the family's annual Fourth of July picnic, the girl and her mother drove north to Camp Ravenswood East in Volo, Illinois. After the girl settled in, she hugged her mother goodbye and turned to a group of girls her own age. Among the unfamiliar faces she would soon find friends who would change her life forever. Meanwhile, her mother drove away from the aging campground thinking, "She won't last the week here."

Days moved quickly and soon the week passed. While the girl had such a great time that she never once even considered calling home, it also never occurred to her that there would be more to this experience than just the one week. At the closing campfire at the end of seven days, the girl was as teary-eyed as the rest of the campers (a group of children as young as 7 and as old as their early 20s), nurses, respiratory therapists, and counselors. The girl's tears were joyful because camp had been so much fun, more than she had ever expected. She had met so many great kids and experienced so many new things. She had set out alone and afraid, yet she had been determined, and so she was not disappointed. Her tears were also mournful. The girl had come to realize the twofold fact that while she would indeed return to camp the following summer, some of her new friends would not be there again because they wouldn't live that long.

"I don't know if I helped any of the kids," the girl said more than once after the summer of 1986, "but they have helped me. I didn't even realize I needed help. And I don't know how I will ever repay them."

As she had promised during the final campfire, the girl went back to camp the next summer and every summer for the next eight years until the camp ceased to exist. And year after year she made new friends only to lose them to cystic fibrosis. The thing that brought them together ultimately tore them from one another. After her college graduation in 1990, she enrolled in a respiratory therapy program at a local university and earned a degree in respiratory care. After graduation, she landed her dream job at Children's Memorial Hospital in Chicago, where many of her friends from camp were treated. Six years later she married a man who also worked as a pediatric respiratory therapist at the same hospital. In 2001 and 2003, she gave birth to beautiful, healthy baby boys. "These are the gifts from the kids who have CF," the girl realizes time and again.

Like cystic fibrosis itself, this story has not ended yet. Rather, it continues, sometimes painfully and always necessarily. This girl's story will not end until a cure for cystic fibrosis is found, and it continues here and now, in this book, because, you see, this girl is . . . me.

Cystic Fibrosis: The Facts

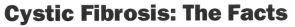

1

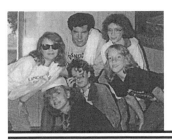

"Do you have CF?" It was a question I had to answer often when I was at cystic fibrosis camp. After all, to some degree I fit the classic picture of someone with cystic fibrosis. At 18, I had just barely reached my full height of five feet and I weighed just ninety-one pounds. Short and thin among my high school friends, I was actually of average height among the girls in my cabin the first year I went to camp. The girls in my cabin ranged in age from 15 to 21 and had just as wide a range in their health. The healthier ones are, after all these years, still alive. The oldest is 40. The other end of the spectrum, the one I was expecting to encounter, was represented as well. Weighing in at just over seventy pounds at five feet two inches tall, Angela Dibbern had just graduated high school, as I had. Angela had plans to attend college. She would finish her freshman year, and with straight As, no less. But cystic fibrosis would take her life a mere fifteen months after I met her, before she could begin her sophomore year of college. Cris, one of the older girls, would live until I was a senior in college, and two others, Lisa and Fonda, would die when we were all in our 20s. The healthiest girls in my cabin, Laura, Jenny, and Sarah*, looked about as healthy as I did (if not more so: Laura was a gymnast) so that comparison was not the giveaway that I did not have CF. I coughed now and then (it rained all week and the cabins were damp) and I had frequent stomach aches (my sensitive stomach was not always pleased with camp food). No, it was not entirely obvious that I did not have cystic fibrosis. The signs and symptoms of cystic fibrosis can be elusive to the untrained eye.

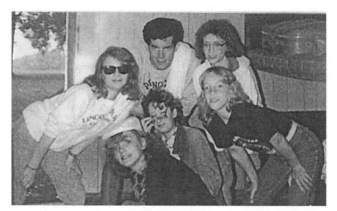

These are the girls in my cabin that first year of camp in 1986. I'm the cool one wearing the shades. In the middle of the top row is a guy named Joe Morrissey who brought his nephew to camp. Aside from Joe and me, of the other four in the photo, Fonda Rae Langston, Cris Shadle, Laura Ballschmeide, and Angela Dibbern, all of whom have CF, only one is still living.

Cystic fibrosis takes the lives of more children and young adults in the United States than any other genetic disease, yet until recently a mention of cystic fibrosis was commonly met with such statements as:

> **Isn't that the thing Jerry Lewis does those telethons for?**
>
> **I think I know someone who had that. He couldn't walk and used a wheelchair.**
>
> **Sixty-five . . . what?!**

Today, with advances in medicine allowing many children who have cystic fibrosis to grow up, there is, necessarily, a new wave of interest in the disease. When asked about cystic fibrosis for the purpose of this book, people from the general population seemed much more aware of the disease than ever.

> "It's a chronic disease that causes thick mucus production mainly in the lungs resulting in coughing, wheezing, and respiratory infections. It's a genetic disorder."—Michele Ottenfeld, 35, Palatine, Illinois

> "Cystic fibrosis is a hereditary disease. Essentially a person with CF has a pair of mutated genes, which means the genes don't

work properly. I first heard about cystic fibrosis in the 1980s after watching a movie based on a true-life story. I believe cystic fibrosis is a cell disorder, which affects the lungs, intestines, and pancreas. Basically sticky, thick mucus is continuously created that destroys the cell tissues in these organs, preventing them from normal human function, such as digestion of food and breathing."—Stephanie Posteau-Gordon, 31 Glenview, Illinois

"There was a movie and book entitled *Alex: The Life of a Child* that I saw in the mid-1980s. I was very moved by it and remember it vividly. This was my first introduction of cystic fibrosis. To my understanding people born with cystic fibrosis produce too much mucus in their lungs, which makes it difficult to breathe. The disease is totally debilitating, affects the very young, and is usually deadly. I think it is genetic."—Samantha Gleisten, 29, Chicago

"When my husband was a student minister in the late 1960s, the minister who he worked for had two sons with cystic fibrosis. Both died in their teens. It's a respiratory disease that causes terrible congestion and affects other body functions as well like the digestive system. Victims have to be 'tapped' every day to try to break up all the thick mucus (at least back then, that was part of the treatment)."—Chloe-Anika Perling*, 54, Chicago

"I first heard of it from my sister-in-law. Also, genetic testing when I was pregnant showed that I was a carrier for cystic fibrosis. It's a genetic disease that affects respiratory systems (among other things). It is a hereditary disease that can be passed on to a child when both parents are carriers."—Judith Glenn*, 36, originally from South Africa

Yet others still remain unclear.

"I have known about cystic fibrosis since 1989 when a friend of my college roommate died of it. But I have no idea what it is. Probably a neuromuscular gene thing."—Kathy French, 33, Arkansas

"I've heard of cystic fibrosis because a cousin of mine was being checked out for potentially having the condition. I'm not sure exactly what it is, but I think it is a condition that someone is born with that impairs their muscles, due to fluid in the lungs. I get it confused with cerebral palsy."—Shonne Fegan-Ehrhardt, 33, Glenview, Illinois

❍

"I have heard of cystic fibrosis from TV. I think it's a condition related to the inflammation of the lungs that you're born with."—Tom, 40, Shonne's husband

❍

"I have heard of cystic fibrosis from telethons and charities but I'm not at all sure what it is. Something with the pancreas I think. I don't know how a person gets cystic fibrosis."—Lana Khawaja, 28, Houston, Texas

❍

"I first heard about cystic fibrosis in 1986, when I was about fifteen years old, from the movie about Alex Deford. Cystic fibrosis is a condition where the lungs do not produce enough moisture or something to keep them . . . well, moist! Mucus builds up causing deterioration of the lungs over time and coughing because it is hard to breathe with full lungs. I know that it affects the absorption of enzymes or something like that, causing people with cystic fibrosis not to be able to absorb their food; hence, they don't gain weight. Lack of oxygen flowing through the system causes clubbing of fingers and toes. A person gets cystic fibrosis when both parents are carriers. Surprising how little I know, considering my sister's eighteen years of involvement with CF, huh?"—Mindy Apel, 32, Chicago, Illinois

❍

"I know of cystic fibrosis because during frosh week at university we did a fund-raising activity called 'shine-a-rama' for a day where we were given a shoe-shining kit to polish the public's shoes for a donation. What I know about cystic fibrosis: genetic disease, problems with respiratory system, lifespan of approximately thirty years, no cure."—Meredith Schaab, 32, Vancouver, BC, Canada

"I've heard of cystic fibrosis from the mailings by the CF Foundation. Isn't it a genetic disease that causes too much mucus to be formed and causes problems with breathing and other body functions? It's inherited, isn't it? Or maybe a genetic disorder—either way, I think a child is born with the disorder."—Alice McGinty, 40, Urbana, Illinois

"I first heard about cystic fibrosis when I was in college. It's sad and scary at the same time. One never knows how the child will be affected by the disease. The closest person I know who has CF is a friend of a friend who has a brother whose child was born with CF. I know that both parents have to carry the 'trait' for the child to have it."—Rhonda Carlson, 35, Chicago

⊚

"I had some contact with Easter Seals (via a friend) and she knew kids with cystic fibrosis. I think it has something to do with mucus membrane . . . buildup of mucus in the nasal cavity. It's hereditary."—Michele Appel, 54, Elgin, Illinois

In 1938 pathologist Dr. Dorothy Anderson of New York's Columbia University made the first pathological description of cystic fibrosis. Reported in the *American Journal of Diseases of Children*, Anderson described an illness that was different from celiac disease, showing how this illness included progressive lung destruction and death in infancy or early childhood. Anderson performed autopsies on infants and children and reviewed their case histories to provide the first comprehensive description of the symptoms of cystic fibrosis and of the damage the disease does to the body's organs. She described how the changes usually included destruction of the pancreas, even in the case of infants, and often infection of and damage to the airways in the lungs. Anderson also named the disease. She called it "cystic fibrosis of the pancreas" because she had found cysts, or fluid-filled sacs, and scar tissue, or fibrosis, in the pancreatic tissue of those she autopsied. These tissues had replaced most of the normal pancreatic tissue. She felt the epithelial changes that she saw in cystic fibrosis were similar to those found in people who suffered from vitamin A deficiency. Therefore, she believed that a vitamin A deficiency was involved in the pathogenesis of CF.[1]

These responses indicate that while the general public is quite aware of cystic fibrosis, their understanding of the disease remains limited. While each of the respondents had heard of cystic fibrosis, and each seemed to have a vague to moderate notion of what it is, very few really knew exactly. Though interestingly they all knew it was hereditary or genetic. Few of those who replied actually know anyone who has CF.

When you finish reading this book, you will have a clear understanding of what cystic fibrosis is and how its symptoms affect a person's body. You will also have some understanding of what it is like to live each day with cystic fibrosis. Reading the stories of children, teens, and adults who live with cystic fibrosis will, hopefully, give you an appreciation for what they go through on a daily basis, as well as an appreciation for your own health if you do not have cystic fibrosis. If you do have CF, probably the most important thing you will learn from this book is that you are not alone.

Although this book covers the broad picture of cystic fibrosis, it is in no way a definitive end-all to the information available about cystic fibrosis. What you will learn here are the basics, and more important you will learn about what it's really like to live with cystic fibrosis. So, while every detail of cystic fibrosis and its treatment cannot possibly be discussed in a book of this scope, you will come away with the big picture. Resources listed throughout and at the end of the book will help you do further research on the various aspects of cystic fibrosis, if you wish to learn more. While the book list might be extensive, the resources available on the Internet are seemingly unlimited.

If you are a person living with cystic fibrosis, this book should stand as an encouraging testimonial to the fact that you are not in this alone. Others out there are facing the same challenges you face every day. Cystic fibrosis might debilitate the body but it does not have to damage the spirit.

In 1955 a child born with cystic fibrosis could be expected to live only about five years. By 1969, a child born with cystic fibrosis could be expected to live roughly fourteen years. By the year 2000, a child born with cystic fibrosis could be given a prognosis of a thirty-two-year lifespan.[2] In 2004, a child born with cystic fibrosis could think about celebrating his or her fortieth birthday. But what is cystic fibrosis, why have these numbers changed so drastically, and what is this disease all about anyway? Soon, you will understand.

WHAT IS CYSTIC FIBROSIS?

If you have read anything at all about cystic fibrosis, it is no secret to you that it has been called the "number one genetic killer of children and young adults in the United States."

Cystic fibrosis is genetic, which means that people who have it are born with it. It is inherited it from both parents. (More on this later.) You cannot catch cystic fibrosis from someone who has it and you can't develop it later in life, although some people defy diagnosis for years. A person who has cystic fibrosis, or CF, suffers from a variety of difficulties affecting a number of his or her organs. The most common symptoms of CF are salty-tasting skin, a chronic cough, wheezing, frequent bouts of pneumonia, a voracious appetite, poor weight gain, and bulky, foul-smelling, greasy stools. In addition, those who have CF have an increased susceptibility to picking up illnesses, and once sick the course of illness is much more serious. For example, when a healthy person gets a cold, he or she might feel poorly for a number of days, might take over-the-counter remedies, and try to carry on as usual. However, when someone who has CF catches a cold, all sorts of medications, additional respiratory treatments, and often hospitalizations become necessary. The common cold for someone who has advanced or end-stage CF can even prove fatal.

All of this happens because the body produces mucus that is abnormally thick and sticky—much more so than the mucus normally produced by a healthy person's body. This mucus causes problems when it gets stuck in the lungs and the pancreas and, in males, the testes. CF severely compromises the three basic requirements to sustain life: breathing, eating, and reproduction.

The Lungs

Healthy lungs produce clear, thin mucus that helps keep them lubricated for easy breathing and helps clean out debris breathed in from the air. The lungs of a person who has CF are filled with thick, sticky mucus, which is difficult to clear from the lungs. This causes a person who has CF to have a chronic cough, which is the body's attempt to clear the lungs. Although annoying to the person who has CF, the cough itself is merely the tip of the iceberg. The mucus also acts as a trap. Dirt, debris, bacteria, and viruses all get stuck in the mucus, causing frequent, damaging lung infections.

The most common lung infection seen in people who have cystic fibrosis is called *Pseudomonas aeruginosa,* which most people just call *Pseudomonas. Pseudomonas* is an opportunistic bacterial infection that, even with today's antibiotics, is hard to clear up. Therefore, once a person has colonized *Pseudomonas* in his or her lungs, it never really goes away. Instead it persists as a low-grade infection that, if given the chance, will flare up and become an infection worthy of a hospital stay. Because *Pseudomonas* makes itself at home in the lungs, it slowly damages them.[3]

After a while (often many years but sometimes just a few), chronic lung infections lead to irreversible lung damage. Damaged lungs obviously do not work as well as healthy lungs; thus, as a person with CF gets older and his or her lungs sustain more and more damage, breathing becomes increasingly

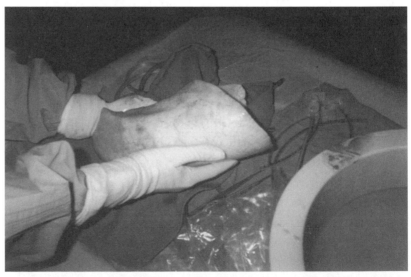

A healthy lower left lobe, inflated and ready to be transplanted into a young lady whose own lungs were damaged by cystic fibrosis.

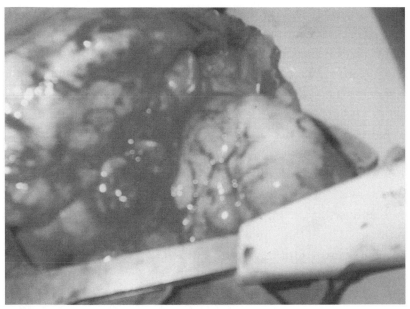

A lung badly damaged by cystic fibrosis. The physician who removed this lung said it resembled bubble wrap.

difficult. Aggressive therapies, which you will read about shortly, help the lungs open and clear, but the effects are only temporary, and a person who has CF will find him- or herself needing to repeat the routine two or more times a day.

Eventually, despite all efforts (and depending on the individual, sometimes sooner and sometimes later), supplemental oxygen will become a necessity. At first oxygen is needed only at night, but then it is needed all day, every day. And despite even this intervention, too much damage and scarring will eventually render the lungs useless, resulting in respiratory failure—and the person essentially suffocates.

Lung damage accounts for more than 90 percent of disability and death of people who have cystic fibrosis. Fortunately, new drugs and new therapies are constantly being tested and prescribed to improve the lung functions of those who have cystic fibrosis.

Digestion

The other main body system affected by the thick, sticky mucus is digestion, specifically the pancreas. Normally, the pancreas produces and secretes enzymes, which help a person's body break down food for digestion, and bicarbonate, which neutralizes stomach acid so the enzymes can work properly in the intestine. With the pancreatic ducts blocked by mucus, the pancreas is unable to send the digestive enzymes out to do their work in the intestines. Thus the nutrition from food does not get absorbed into the body. This pancreatic insufficiency, as it's called, causes people who have CF to have foul-smelling, bulky bowel movements. It also causes malnutrition, slower growth, and slower development. Typically, children who have undiagnosed cystic fibrosis will eat a significantly larger amount of food than their healthy peers, yet they will not gain weight or grow properly because the food literally goes right through them. Often younger, healthy siblings surpass the weight and height of their older sibling who has cystic fibrosis.

Fortunately the body's own natural pancreatic enzymes can be replaced with animal enzyme preparations, which, when taken with meals, allow for virtually normal digestion. The number of enzymes taken before snacks and meals is determined by the doctor and is directly related to age, height, and weight as well as the severity of the person's pancreatic insufficiency.

"I take five enzymes with meals, three with snacks," says Jessica Hawk-Manus.

"I take my four enzymes (Ultrase) with a meal," says Jackie Goryl.

James Lawlor reports taking "five to six Ultrase MT20 with meals, three to five with snacks."

Enzymes come in one preparation: the capsule. Inside each capsule are tiny enzyme beads. This is fortunate for small children who have not yet learned to swallow pills. The capsules can be opened and poured directly into a vehicle of delivery such as applesauce. Four-year-old Betsy Sullivan of San Antonio, Texas, "calls her enzymes birdseed because we open them up and sprinkle them," according to her mom, Mary. Of course, this premeal applesauce every day of your childhood most certainly can lead to a lifelong distaste for applesauce!

Another problem with the pancreas has made its way to the list of CF complications. Because those who have CF are living longer due to better medications, in many indivduals the disease is progressing to a point where cells in the pancreas that make insulin also sustain damage, causing the development of diabetes. Cystic Fibrosis Related Diabetes, or CFRD, is discussed later.

Reproduction

When cystic fibrosis was considered a disease of childhood only, reproduction was not an issue. Today it is. More than 95 percent of men who have CF are sterile. Mucus blocks the testes trapping sperm inside. Another reason men with CF are infertile is that the vas deferens, which carry sperm from the testes, are often either absent or undeveloped. Thankfully, new technologies allow some of these men to become fathers.[4]

Many girls who have cystic fibrosis do not get their first period as early as girls who do not have CF. While her female classmates could, on average, begin getting their periods around age 12 or 13, a girl who has CF might not begin her period until she is closer to 16 or 17 years old. The delay in her onset of puberty is most likely caused by impaired growth overall, a consequence of poor nutrition due to CF.

Some women experience a reduction in their fertility due to abnormal cervical mucus or to menstrual irregularity, but many others have no infertility issues at all. However, doctors have traditionally advised against pregnancy for young women who have cystic fibrosis. Poor lung function and other CF-related issues, such as medications that must be taken to maintain quality of life, might make pregnancy difficult and risky if not physically impossible for some women. Today, many young women who have cystic fibrosis are able to remain relatively healthy with adequate pulmonary function into their 20s, and so with close medical supervision, some have successfully carried pregnancies. It is important to note, however, that a person who has cystic fibrosis has a much greater chance of passing CF to her baby than does a person who is only a CF carrier. You'll read about the genetics of CF in chapter 2.

If you have cystic fibrosis and you are a sexually active teenager or young adult, contraception (birth control) must be considered. While it is true that *most* guys are sterile, this sterility will *only* protect against pregnancy. It does not protect the guy or his partner against acquiring or passing sexually transmitted diseases, including AIDS. Girls who have CF, even if they are not in the best of health, can become pregnant. Whether or not a girl or young woman who has CF should become pregnant is an issue she should discuss with her CF doctor and her gynecologist. The risks she is likely to take with her health might not be worth it, especially if her age and the state of her health will make it difficult for her to care for an infant or child. Any young lady, even those who have CF, can also fall victim to a sexually transmitted disease if she does not use appropriate contraceptives. So whether you are a young man or a young woman who has CF, it is just as important for you as it is for all teens and young adults to take proper precautions to safeguard yourself not only from unplanned pregnancy but also from sexually transmitted diseases. Talk to your CF doctor and get all the facts on safe methods of contraception for those who have CF.

The Rest of the Body

Although the lungs and the pancreas are attacked first and foremost, other parts of the body will eventually begin to feel the effects of cystic fibrosis as well. In addition to providing the body with digestive enzymes, the pancreas is also responsible for making insulin, which breaks down sugars. It is not uncommon for people who have CF to develop Cystic Fibrosis Related Diabetes as early as their late teens. In addition, many people who have CF suffer from sinus trouble and asthma.

Another organ that could sustain serious damage is the liver. In a relatively small number of people who have CF, the bile ducts in the liver are affected, causing biliary cirrhosis. This condition necessitates a liver transplant.

Some people who have CF experience bowel obstructions, collapsed lungs, and other traumatizing setbacks. People who have advanced or end-stage CF will suffer frequent, severe headaches, due to a lack of oxygen and buildup of carbon dioxide in the brain. As CF destroys a person's ability to breathe easily, even with the assistance of supplemental oxygen, a person with CF will lose the desire to eat and, subsequently, the energy to walk or function much at all. At this point, it is inevitable that without intervention, and sometimes even with it, the person with CF will die.

HOW KNOWLEDGE OF CF HAS CHANGED: AN ENCYCLOPEDIA DESCRIPTION OF CYSTIC FIBROSIS, 1963

In 1963, Collier's Encyclopedia included a short article by Harry Shwachman about cystic fibrosis. While the generalization Shwachman made that cystic fibrosis is a "disorder which affects the mucus-secreting glands of the body as well as the external secreting (exocrine) sweat glands" heads in the right direction, it was incorrect in its assumption that CF produces "lesions in various organs, especially the lungs, liver, and pancreas." Back in 1963 it was accurate to print that CF was "primarily a disease of infants and children with few proven adult cases." At the time, it was also accurate to print that "the exact cause" of cystic fibrosis remained "unknown." The encyclopedia entry was correct in its suggestion that the "familial nature of the disease suggests that it is inherited as a Mendelian recessive." However, the postulation at the time was that CF was caused by "a defect in the activity of the mucus glands," which resulted in "abnormally sticky secretions [that] produce duct obstruction with subsequent changes in the affected organs, such as pancreas, lungs, and liver."

Even in 1963 the sweat test was being used to diagnose cystic fibrosis. Collier's article explained that cystic fibrosis "is established by quantitative examination of sweat for chloride and/or sodium. In patients with cystic fibrosis, the average salt content in sweat is from three to five times that found in healthy children. In no other disease is the concentration of salt as high as in cystic fibrosis." The article also goes on to say that "the sweat test appears to be the most useful and reliable diagnostic test at the present time," suggesting that another, more sophisticated method of diagnosis would eventually replace the somewhat primitive sweat test.

Regarding treatment of cystic fibrosis, in 1963 it was standard practice to manage lung involvement with broad-spectrum antibiotics, mist therapy, and "judicious use of iodides," and to manage pancreatic insufficiency with pancreatin capsules taken with meals, along with modifications to the diet that were aimed at reducing total fat intake and "liberal" use of multivitamins. In terms of actual hands-on chest physical therapy, the encyclopedia entry states that "physiotherapy also has much to offer."

Although it admits that CF was primarily a disease of childhood, Collier's was hesitant to give a doomsaying prognosis and says only that "the prognosis varies considerably and depends mostly on the extent and severity of the pulmonary lesion." An encyclopedia entry today would share much more knowledge with its readers. So much has changed—for the better—in forty years.

A normal finger looks like this.

A clubbed finger looks like this.

A healthy fingertip and a clubbed finger tip. Notice how the clubbed finger is rounded and more bulbous than the healthy finger.

While a person who has cystic fibrosis does not look fundamentally different from anyone else, advanced CF can cause some subtle changes to a person's physique. Most notably, people who have CF have some degree of clubbing in their fingers and toes. "When people first meet me," said Kimberlee Pilarczyk, 20, "whether they know I have CF or not, they notice my hands: my clubbed fingernails. That's the first thing. People will go, 'You've got weird fingers.' I just shrug it off."

Clubbed fingers and toes, which can be seen on the hands and feet of most people who have cystic fibrosis, are also known as hypertrophic pulmonary osteoarthropathy. This clubbing, while not a problem itself, is a common side effect of cystic fibrosis. Diseases such as cystic fibrosis in which the heart and lungs are involved, causing chronically low oxygen levels in the blood, often result in clubbing of the fingers and toes. Diseases that cause malabsorption, as do cystic fibrosis and other diseases such as celiac disease, often cause clubbing as well.

Although no one knows for certain why or exactly how the tips of the fingers and toes change shape as CF progresses, it is of interest to note that people who receive lung transplants see a nearly complete reversal of the clubbing. Therefore, it is assumed that clubbing is the result of a lack of oxygen to the finger and toe tips.

Other physical signs of cystic fibrosis are less obvious to the untrained eye. Some people who have cystic fibrosis have a rounded or "barrel" shaped rib cage and chest. Some have a rounded, protruding belly. In years past, due to inadequate

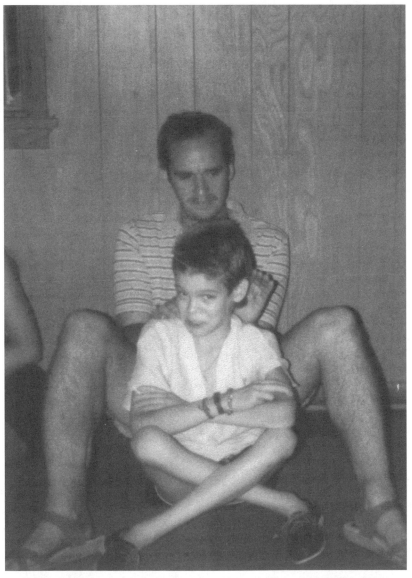

Troy Morrison was a classic picture of cystic fibrosis in 1986. Thin and shorter than average at 14 years old, Troy, shown getting therapy at camp, died less than three months after this photo was taken.

nutrition, most children and teens who had CF were shorter in stature and significantly thinner than their peers. Today, thanks to medical interventions (which are discussed in a later chapter), these physical differences are not as apparent until end-stage CF and even then not in all people who have CF. Finally, people who have CF might appear pale, due to lack of sufficient oxygen.

Before I had my lung transplant my sister always said I looked blue, like skim milk. —Amy Thom, 19

Oh, this is such a grim picture! Fortunately, however, this is no longer an accurate portrayal of the whole life of a person who has cystic fibrosis. Rather, this is the picture of cystic fibrosis if left untreated (or of end-stage cystic fibrosis). You can see why most children did not live long before cystic fibrosis was understood by the medical profession. Today, thanks to research and wonderful medical breakthroughs, the true picture of a person living with CF is often much brighter. In fact, eighteen years ago typical symptoms of cystic fibrosis, such as clubbed fingers and toes, shorter-than-average stature, pale skin, and extreme thinness, could have been attributed to even the youngest children with CF. Today, until the disease progresses quite far, a person

Did You Know?
Some small children who have cystic fibrosis think their disease is called sixty-five roses.

with CF can look as healthy as his or her peers and lead an active, healthy life for many years.

RECAP OF SYMPTOMS

So, to recap, the symptoms that cause suspicion of cystic fibrosis include:

- Persistent cough sometimes producing mucus
- Recurrent wheezing or breathing difficulty
- Recurrent pneumonia
- Frequent sinus and respiratory infections
- Frequent foul-smelling, bulky stools and chronic diarrhea
- Good appetite but poor body growth and weight gain
- Nasal polyps (bumps inside the nose)
- Enlarged fingertips and toe tips (clubbing)
- Skin that is salty to the taste
- Sterility in males[5]

Did You Know?
- There are many different gene mutations that cause CF.
- The mutations one carries for CF do not necessarily determine the CF symptoms one will exhibit.
- Some people with CF do not need to take enzymes.
- Some people with CF are "overweight."
- Some people with CF are diagnosed late in life.[6]

BUT WHY? AND HOW?

Cystic fibrosis is caused by a gene mutation or, more accurately, a pair of gene mutations, one from each parent. Because of these mutations the normal function of epithelial cells is disrupted. Epithelial cells line the passageways in the lungs, liver, pancreas, and digestive and reproductive systems, and make up the sweat glands in the skin. The CF gene tells the epithelial cells to produce a defective form of a specific protein. This protein, called CFTR (cystic fibrosis transmembrane conductance regulator), when defective, causes the epithelial cells to lose their ability to regulate the way chloride passes across cell membranes. Chloride is part of the salt called sodium chloride. When the chloride cannot pass freely, the essential balance of salt and water in the body necessary for maintaining the normal, thin coating of fluid and mucus inside the lungs, pancreas, and passageways in other organs is disrupted. Instead of healthy, thin mucus, the mucus becomes thick and sticky. It does not move easily through the body.[7]

Humans have forty-six chromosomes or twenty-three pairs. One chromosome of each pair is inherited from each parent. It is now known that the gene that causes cystic fibrosis is found on the long arm of chromosome number 7. Scientists have been able to identify more than 850 different mutations of the CF gene. Accounting for roughly 90 percent of all cases of cystic fibrosis is a mutation named Delta F508. The gene that causes CF can be found through genetic testing, which is available to adults, children, and unborn babies.[8]

BOYS VERSUS GIRLS IN THE GAME OF LIFE

For reasons not clearly understood by medical professionals, cystic fibrosis tends to be harder on teenage girls and women than it is on their male counterparts. Hormones are suspected to play a role in this discrepancy, especially when taken into consideration around the female menstrual cycle. Males might also respond better to certain medications. In the "old" days of cystic fibrosis, when it was more typical to find a little boy outside playing baseball and a little girl indoors playing with her dolls, the odds were stacked even more in favor of the boys,

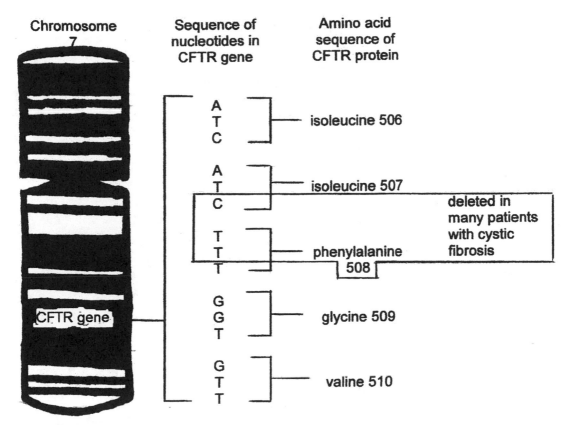

| Chromosome 7 | Sequence of nucleotides in CFTR gene | Amino acid sequence of CFTR protein |

Chromosome 7. The gene that is responsible for causing cystic fibrosis is found on chromosome 7. Normally—that is, in people who do not have cystic fibrosis—this gene gives rise to a protein called the cystic fibrosis transmembrane conductance regulator (CFTR). In the person who has cystic fibrosis, the CFTR does not work properly. The defect that most often leads to cystic fibrosis is known as the Delta F508 mutation. This mutation is caused by the deletion of three nucleotides from the gene, as noted in the diagram. The mutation causes phenylalanine at position 508 to be lost from the CFTR protein because the protein-making machinery of the cell now sees "ATT," which is an alternative way to encode isoleucine at the gene region coding for amino acid number 507 on the protein. Next it sees the GGT sequence for the glycine that should normally follow phenylalanine. Without the phenylalanine at position 508, the entire sequence is "messed up" and cystic fibrosis results.

as their natural tendency toward a more physical lifestyle worked well to strengthen their lungs, thus helping them stay healthier for a longer period of time overall. Today, however, much more is understood about the role of exercise in maintaining good lung function, and so both boys and girls are encouraged to try physical activities such as team sports, gymnastics, martial arts, dance, and even playing a musical instrument. (You'll read more about CF and exercise later.)

ANOTHER BOOK WORTH READING

Robyn's Book: A True Story by Robyn Miller (New York: Scholastic, 1986) is a 21-year-old girl's account of life with cystic fibrosis. Although the book was written in the 1980s and medical advances have changed certain aspects of CF, Robyn's feelings about living with the disease, and losing friends to the disease, are still valid today.

NOTES

1. Jim Littlewood, "The Historical Development of Nutritional and Dietetic Management of Cystic Fibrosis," April 2002, www.sustainit.com/cfmain/open/topics/CFTest/historydiet.html.

2. Norma Kennedy Plourde's Cystic Fibrosis website, personal .nbnet.nb.ca/nnormap/CF.htm, or www3.nbnet.nb.ca/normap/cfhistory.htm.

3. NIDDK: Cystic fibrosis research directions, www.niddk.nih .gov.health/endo/pubs/cystic/cystic.htm.

4. Cystic Fibrosis Foundation, cff.org/about_cf/what_is_cf .cfm?CFID=1619012&CFTOKEN=84991526.

5. Arizona Respiratory Center, www.resp-sci.arizona.edu/ patient-info/child/cystic-fibrosis-k.htm.

6. Anne Keator, Rochester, New York, e-mail message to author, February 2003.

7. Kids Health for Parents, websrv02.kidshealth.org/parent/medical/digestive/cf.html.

8. Kids Health for Parents.

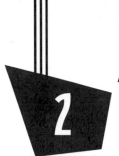

A Genetic Disorder

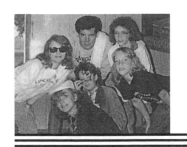

Cystic fibrosis is an autosomal, recessive, genetically inherited disease. Whew! What does *that* mean? Let's see . . .

TWO CARRIERS

"We had no idea we were CF carriers." This quote could be attributed to just about any parent who, for the first time, experiences the birth of a child who has cystic fibrosis. "My mom remembers being told about an aunt who was much older than she was. She was skinny and she coughed a lot. And she died when she was young. But no one had ever mentioned cystic fibrosis. My dad had an uncle who died young, too, but again, no one had ever heard of cystic fibrosis," said Kimberlee Pilarczyk about her family's surprise upon learning that she had cystic fibrosis, especially because her parents had already given birth to a healthy child before her. Kimberlee's older sister does not have cystic fibrosis.

Did You Know?
Mackenzie Rosman, who plays Ruthie Camden on the WB's *7th Heaven*, has a stepsister who has CF.

Less than two months after I spent my first week at cystic fibrosis camp, I packed my belongings and headed for college to begin my freshman year. With my week at camp still in the forefront of my mind, I spoke of it often. I even enrolled in a human genetics course during my first semester. I thought it would help me to better understand cystic fibrosis and how it is inherited. Maybe it would help me understand why I had all these new friends who were so desperately sick with cystic fibrosis.

Without actually producing a child who has cystic fibrosis, or having a genetic test to determine carrier status, there is no way to know whether a person might carry the gene that causes cystic fibrosis. Until quite recently, the only way people found out that they were CF carriers was when they actually gave birth to a child who had CF. Of course, the way genetics work and the way the odds run, there are many people, even those who have children, who never know they are CF carriers. This is confusing.

A GENETICS LESSON

For a child to be born with cystic fibrosis, both parents have to be carriers of the CF gene. One carrier parent paired with one noncarrier parent *cannot* produce a child who has CF. However, the carrier parent paired with the noncarrier parent *can* produce carrier children.

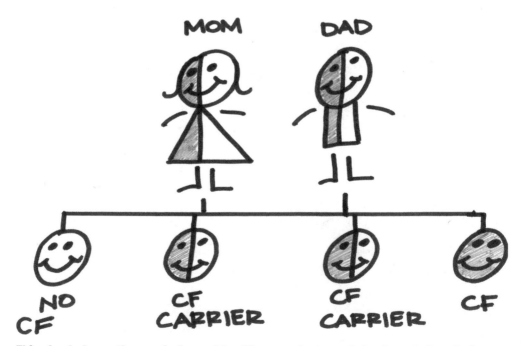

This chart shows the one-in-four odds of two carrier parents having a baby who has cystic fibrosis, the two-in-four odds of having a baby who is a carrier, and the one-in-four odds that their baby will have no CF gene at all.

For two carrier parents the odds of having a child who has CF are high: 25 percent. That's a one-in-four chance. The odds of the two carrier parents having a child who is a carrier are 50 percent, or two in four. The best-case scenario also has one-in-four odds: no CF and no chance of passing down CF, 25 percent. These odds were once explained another way, which might seem somewhat clearer but is also less accurate: if two carrier parents produce four children, one will have CF, two will be carriers, and one will be completely unaffected. While this gives a statistical picture that is easy to understand, it does not really give an accurate picture. If it did, the chances of having more than one child with CF would only be something to worry about if the parents were planning to have more than four children. The reality of the odds is that *each* pregnancy has a 25 percent chance of producing a child who has CF. The odds of having a healthy child are a high 75 percent. The 25 percent chance of having a child who has CF might not look so high in comparison but, in fact, 25 percent is actually a significant chance. Would you take the chance? It can be a tough call for many parents after they have one child who has cystic fibrosis.

"We had two and two," said Mike DiBiase. "My sister Jenny and I were born with CF. My brother Ken and my sister Christin were not. I don't know whether or not they are carriers." Most siblings of kids who have CF will get tested to see if they are carriers before they have children of their own.

"I don't know if I am a carrier," says Craig Lucci. "But when I get married I will get tested. If I am a carrier, I will have my wife tested to see if she is, too." Craig is the elder of two boys. His younger brother Chad has CF.

Plenty of families have multiple healthy children and only one child who has cystic fibrosis. In some families two, three, or even more children have CF. In other families all of the children have CF. Many parents opt not to have any more children once they have one who has CF. For them, the 25 percent chance of having another child who has cystic fibrosis is too much of a risk. Others have more than one child who has cystic fibrosis only because they were unaware of the first case of CF before they had more children.

"My parents didn't know I had CF when I was really little. My brother Ken was healthy, and I seemed healthy enough. Then my sister Jenny was born and she was sick right from the beginning. When she was diagnosed with CF the doctor said that my brother and I had to be tested. Ken was healthy. My parents were pretty surprised to find out that I had CF, too. My sister Christin is a lot younger than Jenny. Maybe my parents had to really think about whether or not they wanted to risk having three kids with CF. Luckily Christin doesn't have CF."—Mike DiBiase

"We took the chance. After Maggie was diagnosed, we thought long and hard about whether or not to have more children. We knew that to do so would be playing a genetic game of Russian roulette. But we wanted two children and we felt the 25 percent chance of having another with CF was low enough odds for us. Our son Steven was born when Maggie was three and he doesn't have CF."—Kerry Sheehan

WHO ARE THE CARRIERS?

While it is not known precisely how many people in the world have cystic fibrosis, it is estimated that between 70,000 and 100,000 people worldwide have the disease. It is likely, however, that many more people have it than have been reported. About 30,000 children and adults who have cystic fibrosis live in the United States. This is a fairly large number. Yet it would almost seem as if more people in the United States would have CF, considering the fact that one out of every 31 Americans, or 5 percent of the population, is a carrier of the gene that causes CF. This statistic can be broken down even further to say that one out of every 28 Caucasians in the United States is a carrier. How many people is that altogether? Roughly ten million!

On average, one in every 3,300 Caucasian babies is born with cystic fibrosis every year in the United States. One thousand new diagnoses are made in the United States every year.[1] While Caucasians have the highest incidence of CF, it is found in other ethnic groupings as well. At one time, it was believed that only the Caucasian population, especially those with family roots in eastern Europe, carried the gene that causes CF. Today, however, because of easy travel and interracial families, almost every ethnic and racial group has a chance of producing children who have CF. The incidence of CF births drops dramatically in the African American population, with one CF birth out of every 17,000 African American births. The Asian American population sees the lowest incidence with only one CF birth in every 90,000 Asian American births. CF has been noted in every part of the world among every ethnic population.[2] Approximately 3,000 children and adults who have cystic fibrosis live in Canada.

Those who carry the gene that causes cystic fibrosis have no symptoms of cystic fibrosis. But their cells carry a single mutant version of the gene. Cystic fibrosis remains one of the most common genetic diseases in the United States.[3] Most people who have CF, more than 80 percent in fact, are diagnosed by the time they are three years old. Surprisingly, however, almost 10 percent are diagnosed when they are 18 years old or older.[5]

Did You Know?
While most cases of CF are caused by the Delta F508 mutation, there are more than 1,000 mutations of the CF gene, which might account for the variations in the disease from one person to the next.[4]

From what I knew of cystic fibrosis at the time I first went to CF camp in 1986, only white children had it. You can imagine my surprise at finding a couple of African American kids at camp. Later, after I became a respiratory therapist, I worked for six years at Children's Memorial Hospital in Chicago. During that time the "whites only" theory was blown out of the water as I not only took care of more and more African American kids, but I also treated a fair share of Hispanic kids, plus an Indian boy with cystic fibrosis (although I can no longer remember the exact theory behind the origin of his CF). Also, as there were only two Jewish families at camp, I was very surprised to learn that a Jewish ancestry is now considered a higher risk for carrying the CF gene. Oh, but to take the

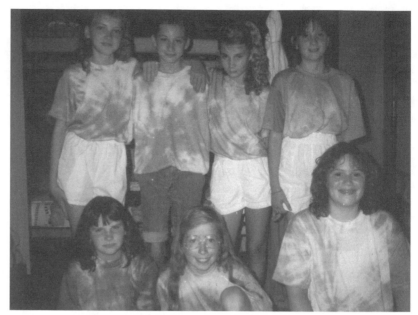

Of the seven girls pictured in this cabin group (front row: Angela Budnieski, Kelly Hutchings, Emily Rose; back row: Amy Thom, Brandy Miller, Cassondra Ditzler, Jessica Denny), only Emily did not have CF. You can read about Amy and Angela later in this book. None of the six campers with CF in this photo lived to see her 30th birthday.

"white" theory to a crazy extreme, my mom will tell you that (based on the friends of mine from CF camp whom she met) all kids with CF have blonde hair!

So the odds are there. The genetics are simple to understand. And like the lottery itself, it's all a matter of chance.

ANOTHER BOOK WORTH READING

Cystic fibrosis and DNA are the subjects in Syne Mitchell's science fiction work *The Changeling Plague* (New York: Roc, 2003). A man who has cystic fibrosis and also happens to be a millionaire injects himself with an experimental virus in the hopes of reprogramming his body's DNA to free himself from cystic fibrosis. Instead of changing just his own life, however, he changes the DNA of everyone around him thus making way for a global disaster of new and strange diseases and deformities.

WHY?

You might be asking yourself a seemingly simple question right about now: *Why?* Why would a devastating disease such as cystic fibrosis exist at all? While it might seem like an answer to this question would be elusive, in fact here it is. Researchers at Harvard University along with researchers at England's Cambridge University and Bristol University believe they've found the reason for the existence of cystic fibrosis. Their research led them to the belief that people who have just one single copy of the mutated gene are protected against infection by the bacterium that causes typhoid. Typhoid is an illness uncommon in developed countries today. A person living in areas with poor sanitation is most likely to get typhoid from eating food or drinking water contaminated with a bacterium called *Salmonella typhi*. The *Salmonella typhi* travels on infected food and water into the digestive system. It then makes its way into the intestinal wall and on into the bloodstream. People who carry one copy of the mutated CFTR gene gain protection against such infection.

Inside these carriers' lungs, a protein that is produced by the CFTR gene binds to another bacterium, usually *Pseudomonas aeruginosa*, and causes the germ to be expelled by coughing, sneezing, or expectoration. People who have cystic fibrosis carry two copies of the mutated CFTR gene and are not protected from typhoid or any other disease. In fact, it is the cystic fibrosis patients' lack of this specific protector protein that causes them to suffer infections that clog their airways and destroy their lung tissue.[6]

PROGNOSIS

The prognosis for someone who has cystic fibrosis can be as individualized as the person. Today, the median age of life expectancy for a person with CF is 35.1 years. Since this is the median age, there are many who live longer and many who live shorter lives than this. For the baby born with cystic fibrosis today, however, a life expectancy of approximately 40 years is reasonable to assume. Yet some don't make it very long at all and others fly past the statistical age as if it were merely an arbitrary number. Prognosis is based on many factors including (but not limited to) age at diagnosis and damage already done by the time of diagnosis. A prognosis is in no way a law set in stone because the truth is, one just never knows.

> "When I was diagnosed at age 12, in 1956, the life expectancy for children with CF was about four years of age. My parents were told to take me home and 'enjoy' me because I wouldn't live six months. Today, *forty-eight years later*, I still am living and functioning quite well. All of the docs who cared for me then are dead!"—Kathy Russell, Gresham, Oregon

Kathy is 60 years old. Kathy's story might not be typical but it is inspirational and it shows that doctors are not clairvoyant.

> "I was not expected to make it to kindergarten. I made it to kindergarten and they said I wouldn't make it to high school. I made it to high school and they thought I wouldn't make it out. I did. I am now 23, and I'm still kicking and doing great."
> —Jennifer Cherry

Laura Tillman of Northville, Michigan, was diagnosed with cystic fibrosis as an adult, which is in defiance of the odds in and of itself:

> "When I was diagnosed I had already beaten the odds by forty-six years," says Laura. "My life expectancy was one year. But my diagnosis came at 47 years of age. I'll be 57 on December 22, 2004. I just continue defying those numbers!"

A more typical story comes from Brenda Morey of Placentia, California:

> "When my daughter Angela was diagnosed in 1984 the docs said she had a 50/50 chance of living to be 18. She is 20 now and doing well. I know a lot of people who are Angela's age who did not live to be 18, but we are not related to any of them."

And of course there are those who hit the median age right on:

"When [my daughter] Sarah was born in 1981, they said that the median age for CF patients was 21. She died when she was 21," says Sam Feinstein of Bridgeton, New Jersey, whose daughter died on December 21, 2002.

In September 2004, Cara Steading, 18, of San Antonio, Texas, wrote about meeting her new stepbrother, Rodney, for the first time and then losing him to cystic fibrosis a short time later.

RODNEY

I look down. There he is. He's so small. I love his little cheeks. They're the color of pink carnations. His eyes shimmer with excitement. He says, "Hello," and I hear the 'bama accent ring through his voice. I notice the tube running from his backpack up into his nose, and I get nervous. If I give him a hug will I squeeze too hard? What if he doesn't want me to hug him? Maybe I should shake his hand? What am I talking about? This is crazy. Leaning down, I wrap my arms around his little body. I feel his heartbeat strum against my chest. My first time ever to hug my stepbrother.

We sit in the backseat and I hear the faint whisper of country on the radio. I see my dad's shaggy beard in the rearview mirror. His smile is hidden beneath it. I feel Rodney's gaze on me, but I look out the window. I don't know what to say. A sign says we're now in Gadson City. We pull into a seafood restaurant called Top O' the River. I wonder how Alabama seafood is. They don't have an ocean anywhere nearby. Inside we sit down at one of the booths. Menus and silverware are laid in front of us. For the first time I get a good look at Sherrie, my new stepmom. Highlighted blonde hair frames her tan face. Her eyes are warm and caring, and I see a hint of sadness in their depths. Her voice is soft, and there's the same Alabama accent as Rodney's. Now I see why my dad left Austin for a lady he had met only once before. This country girl has my dad wrapped around her little finger with that sweet accent of hers. I smile, watching the two of them exchange kisses throughout the meal. The waitress comes and I order shrimp, considering shrimp can still taste the same after twenty-four hours of shipping and handling.

(*continued*)

Although it's dark out, I know when we've reached their house. It's much prettier than in the pictures. It reminds me of a perfect country home with its white wooden walls, big windows, and giant front porch. I imagine the three of them lounging in rocking chairs, drinking iced tea on hot afternoons. I get the sudden urge to run up and kiss the house and its sweetness. Instead we go inside where I'm given a short tour around. Rodney nearly jumps out of his skin with excitement when we finally head up the stairs to his room. He jets back and forth and I get out of breath just watching him. He shows me his swords, the figurines hung on his wall, his stuffed animals, his video game collection, his games, and his swords one more time. Sherrie comes in and herds Rodney over to the bed. He sits on the edge and she puts a vest over him. Switching it on, the room fills with a loud buzzing noise. I watch as Rodney's body shakes from head to toe from the powerful vibrating. I feel uncomfortable standing in his room watching this, so I start to drift toward the stairs. Glancing back I say a swift "goodnight" and start to head down the stairs. "I love you sis!" Rodney calls after me. My hand grasps the handrail, and I look up. "I love you too, Rod," I call back to him. I can hear them talking and laughing above me.

The sun glares through my window in the morning, toasting my face. I slide my feet around under the covers, loving the feeling of the silk sheets. Even my pillow is silk and I rub my cheek across it. Soon the sun becomes unbearable so I slip out of bed and head for the kitchen. I pour myself some juice and sit down at the dining room table.

"Well, good morning sleepyhead," my dad says from the doorway. "We were wondering if you were going to wake up today or not. Rodney's driving me nuts asking every five minutes when you're going to get up."

Right then Rodney hustles past my dad and comes and sits next to me. I ruffle his hair and grin at him. "What you got planned for us today Rodney?" I ask.

"I want to show you my new video games. This one game is really cool; you have to shoot all of these Zombies. We can watch a movie, too, if you want."

My juice is still half full when I'm tugged upstairs to go shoot at Zombies. Rodney laughs when I shoot at my own men or when I die after only a few seconds. When I die from falling off a ledge his laughing turns to wheezing and then to a terrible cough. I can hear his lungs trying to rid themselves of all the fluid. My hands fidget on my lap, and I feel helpless. Finally his coughing ceases, leaving his face pink from the effort. He turns off the Nintendo and slowly makes his way downstairs. We go in to the living room and watch an old soap opera on TV. I don't know why neither of us changes the channel. "Sis, is there anything you want in my room when I die?" Rodney asks, gazing at me from across the room. I wonder if he can hear my heart thundering. "No, no, I don't think so," I reply weakly. I stare at the VCR. I can't blink. My heart hurts.

Being home feels good, but I miss the three of them already. I talk to Rodney constantly over the Internet, or when my dad calls he'll give him the phone.

"I love you, Sis. I miss you. When are you coming back to visit?" he asks me repeatedly. I smile and tell him, "Soon I hope. I miss you so much."

My dad calls too soon after that and tells me Rodney isn't doing well. My heart drops down to the pit of my stomach. I have to force air into my lungs. "We asked him what he wished for more than anything, and he told us that he wants to see his sister one more time before he dies." There's silence. "I know that would be really hard on you, but I think you can handle it. You're a strong girl, and it would mean the world to him if you'd come."

Sitting on the plane going to see my stepbrother one last time is a heart-wrenching experience. We play video games, and he lets me win. We watch movies in complete silence. Sherrie and my dad buy a cake and we celebrate his 12th birthday early. He slowly unwraps his presents and sets them to the side. We all eat dinner together, but Rodney doesn't eat. Although I'm here, in his home, I barely see him. He sleeps away the days, coughing constantly, morning and night. The illness owns him, has taken over his little body, and there's nothing we can do to help.

"I love you Rodney."

I lean down and hug him. I say goodbye to Sherrie and my dad and get on the plane to head back home. Tears run down my face as I watch the airport drift out of sight. It's tough to go see your dying stepbrother, but it's much worse to say goodbye.

Sitting at the computer, about to go online, my mom walks in. I let go of the mouse and look at her. Something feels wrong. She leans against the edge of the doorway, her gaze lingering a little past my right shoulder. A frown tugs at the corner of her lips. I wait in silence, giving her time to gather her words for what she is going to tell me. Her lips move.

(continued)

"Rodney died last night. Your dad called a while ago, while you were at the store. He said he'll call you again later and that he loves you."

I have just been punched in the stomach. My body crumples up in a ball, and sobs rack through me. I can't feel my mom's hand rubbing my back. My head shakes back and forth. No, no, no, NO. This does not happen. He does not leave like this. I refuse for this to happen.

I lie in bed with the blankets pulled up to my neck. My eyes close and there he is, waiting for me beneath my eyelids. Tears blur his image. Don't worry little brother, I have a plan that will change everything. I'm going to pick up my remote and rewind to the day I first saw you, with your eyes full of excitement. I'm going to take you to carnivals and fancy restaurants, and we'll go and buy tons of video games and play them all night long. I'll take you to museums where swords are encased in glass. I'm going to show you the world, Rodney, because you deserve to see it. You love me and you don't even know me. You love me because I'm your sister, and you don't care about anything else. You don't care what I look like, or that I'm really bad at video games, or that my heart isn't as big as yours. I'll take you to the best doctor in the world Rodney, even if he's on the other side of the world. We're going to walk into his office and he's going to smile. It's our lucky day! He has just discovered the cure for cystic fibrosis! We're going back to the little white country house in Piedmont. The four of us are going to sit on that huge front porch and drink iced tea, even if it's cold outside. This is what will happen when I press the rewind, Rodney, because I don't think I can handle this ending. I close my eyes and there you are, just beneath my eyelids. Where would you like to go, little Rodney? We have so little time before I wake up.

—Cara Steading, September 13, 2004

NOTES

1. Cystic Fibrosis Foundation, cff.org/about_cf/what_is_cf .cfm?CFID=1619012&CFTOKEN=84991526.

2. Kids Health for Parents, websrv02.kidshealth.org/parent/ medical/digestive/cf.html.

3. Norma Kennedy Plourde's Cystic Fibrosis website, personal .nbnet.nb.ca/nnormap/CF.htm, or www3.nbnet.nb.ca/normap/ cfhistory.htm.

4. Cystic Fibrosis Foundation.

5. Cystic Fibrosis Foundation.

6. William J. Cromie, "Cystic Fibrosis Gene Found to Protect Against Typhoid," Gazette staff, www.hno.harvard.edu/gazette/1998/07.09/CysticFibrosisG.html.

A Diagnosis

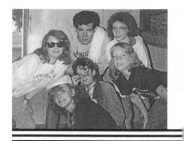

3

> "I was diagnosed right at birth. I had a surgery for meconium ileus at one day old. I had another surgery exactly a month later to help reconstruct my intestines," says Jessica Hawk-Manus.

Healthy babies have their first bowel movement within the first twenty-four hours after they are born. This first bowel movement consists of a sticky, black, tarlike substance called meconium. Newborns will have several of these bowel movements within the first few days of life until the meconium is eliminated from their bowels and their normal stools develop. Roughly 15 percent of babies born with CF are born with a condition called meconium ileus in which the meconium remains blocked within the bowel. When the meconium does not come out within the first twenty-four hours, cystic fibrosis is suspected. A baby born with meconium ileus will automatically be given a sweat test to confirm a diagnosis of cystic fibrosis.

Meconium ileus is such a serious problem for the newborn, it is actually life threatening. Surgery within a few hours is usually necessary. Without surgery the baby will be unable to pass the stool and will suffer a ruptured bowel. He or she will

There was a little girl named Andrea who came to CF camp for a few years. "We had no idea she had CF," I remember her mom saying. "She had asthma and stomach problems, but her doctor never put the two together." While many babies are diagnosed with cystic fibrosis immediately following their birth because they present with a problem called meconium ileus, other children defy a diagnosis for months or even years for one reason or another.

35

die as a result. The baby might require an ostomy, or opening in the bowel through the belly, following the surgery to clear the obstruction. The ostomy allows the traumatized bowel to heal properly for a time, often several months, so that it can eventually function properly. On occasion, meconium ileus develops several months *before* the baby is born and can be seen during a routine ultrasound of the pregnant mother's belly. This situation is called Bright Bowel or Echogenic Bowel and is a strong indication that the baby will be born with cystic fibrosis. When this occurs, the mother will be advised to consult with a CF specialist to discuss her options, weighing the risks of her baby's bowel distending in utero until it possibly ruptures versus allowing the baby to be born early to avoid rupture but then not allowing the baby's lungs to mature fully.[1]

Dawn Pontious, a mother in Lexington, South Carolina, experienced meconium ileus with her son Tyler, who is now 6 years old.

SAVING TYLER

"My son, Tyler, was born at 38½ weeks gestation via C-section after nineteen hours of labor. When they took him out, his belly was very distended, red, and swollen. When he was five hours old they did exploratory surgery to find out what the problem was and they found that he'd had a blockage and that it had ruptured in utero. They cut out a portion of his intestine and gave him an ostomy to give his intestines five weeks to heal. They told me they weren't sure if his lower intestines would ever work because they had never been stimulated. When Tyler was five weeks old, they reconnected his intestines and we waited for his first bowel movement (BM). With the help of suppositories to help stimulate the lower portion of his intestines, and after a few days (maybe a week), he finally had a BM. They told us that Tyler was very lucky to have made it because he was badly infected from the rupture. Looking back on my pregnancy, we might have realized that something was wrong when at thirty-three weeks pregnant I was measuring around thirty-six weeks. So I think it must have been around thirty-one weeks, or maybe even earlier than that, when Tyler's intestines started to get blocked up. I was scheduled for an ultrasound at 38½ weeks, but the night before the appointment, my water broke and Tyler was born the next day. I'm very glad that happened; otherwise, Tyler might not be here today."

THE TYPICAL DIAGNOSIS: THE SWEAT TEST

While some babies are diagnosed right away because they present with meconium ileus, others are diagnosed later for different reasons, but usually still within the first two years of life. "When I was 2 years old my grandmother heard a program on the radio about CF and realized that I had all the symptoms, so she told my mother to have me tested," says 19-year-old Alice Vosloo of Port Elizabeth, South Africa.

Because people who have CF have an increased amount of salt in their sweat, cystic fibrosis is most commonly diagnosed with a simple and even somewhat primitive test, called a sweat test. A sweat test is performed on any baby, child, or adult who is suspected of having cystic fibrosis, despite the symptoms. In other words, even if a child shows all of the symptoms of CF, he or she will still be given a sweat test for confirmation of the disease.

There's an old German folk saying: "The baby who is kissed at birth and tastes salty will have a short life." This illustrates that cystic fibrosis was around long before it had a name.

"I had a sweat test and was diagnosed in 1982 at about six months of age," says Jackie Goryl, 23, of Kalamazoo, Michigan.

The sweat test has been used to diagnose cystic fibrosis for more than forty years.[2] When a person is exhibiting classic signs of cystic fibrosis, such as recurring respiratory illness and malabsorption of foods, or if there is suspected cystic fibrosis due to a family history of CF, a sweat test is used to confirm a diagnosis. The sweat test measures the amount of salt, or sodium chloride, in the sweat. To perform a sweat test, a solution using a chemical called pilocarpine, which is known to enhance sweating, is rubbed on a small spot on each arm. Electrodes, which release a mild and painless electric current, are attached to these spots, stimulating the skin to sweat. Some people describe the feeling of the electrodes as a tingling, a mild discomfort, or warmness. After about five minutes, gauze pads and plastic wrap are wrapped around the stimulated areas. The sweat is collected on the gauze pads over a period of approximately thirty minutes, during which time the child can generally resume regular activities while waiting. The sweat is analyzed in a lab.[3]

The sweat test has been used to test for cystic fibrosis since 1953.

If the level of salt in the sweat is higher than normal, that is, if it is above 60 mmol/L (60 mEq/L)[4] a diagnosis of CF is made. (Mmol/L means millimoles per liter and mEq/L means millequivalents per liter.) On occasion, a sweat test might have a borderline result, that is, one in which the salt level falls between 40 and 60 mmol/L. It is not within the normal range, but is not so high out of range as to confirm a diagnosis.[5] In cases such as this the sweat test can be repeated several times. Today, genetic testing and other diagnostic tools are helpful in confirming a diagnosis.[6]

While people who have cystic fibrosis have more salt in their sweat than normal, they do not sweat any more than other people.[7]

ADDITIONAL TESTS CAN CONFIRM DIAGNOSIS

Cells scraped from the inside of the cheek can be tested for mutations in the CFTR gene. Blood tests can detect infections and possible involvement of certain organs. Chest X-rays can be used to look for lung damage. Pulmonary function tests, or PFTs, measure the lungs' ability to properly exchange oxygen and carbon dioxide. PFTs are done in a dedicated PFT lab with special machines that one breathes into, following specific directions. PFTs are not useful for diagnosing infants or very young children. Sputum cultures can be performed on the mucus that is coughed up from the lungs and spit out. Sputum cultures are also valuable in diagnosing lung infections.[8]

In addition to the hallmark respiratory symptoms of cystic fibrosis, another telltale sign that a person has CF is that his or her stools are abnormal. Usually the parent of a child with CF will notice that the child makes frequent trips to the bathroom and that the results are a floating, bulky, greasy, foul-smelling mess. Subsequently, the child is thin and small for his or her age, despite the fact that he or she might be the most voracious eater in the family. The child's stool sample can be taken to assist in the diagnosis of CF. The stool sample is tested to measure how much fat it contains. High fat content in the stool indicates that the fat is being eliminated from the body rather than being absorbed properly.

DIAGNOSING MAGGIE

"For the first year of Maggie's life I thought she was fine," explains Kerry Sheehan, mom of 15-year-old Maggie. "I thought her spitting up and coughing was probably an allergy or something. I knew she was tiny for her age, but my husband and I are no giants. We had no reason to think she was sick. She coughed in the isolette in the nursery right after she was born. But again, I just remember my sister saying, 'Isn't that cute to see a baby cough?' It's like when they sneeze and it looks so adorable. Even then, they checked her throat, but they said everything was okay.

"We were doing a modeling thing the day we found out Maggie has CF. She was going to get a permit to model, which requires, among other things, a doctor's okay. We had already told the doctor countless times that Maggie had been spitting up a lot and that she was always coughing. He could never find anything wrong. Then that day we went to get the permit the doctor saw her cough and spit up. He said, 'What's that?' I said, 'That's what she has been doing.' And that's when he said, 'Let's do a sweat test,' and sent us over to Loyola Medical Center.

"The day she turned 13 months old, from the moment she was diagnosed, it was just like 'BOOM!' Everything was a whirlwind. I'll never forget. . . . It was a lab guy who was reading the results and he was saying, 'Yeah, well, I've only had one positive in the two years I've worked here, and so it's highly unlikely, but we have to rule it out.' Then he said that most of the time babies with CF taste salty. As soon as he said that I knew! I had remembered nursing her the summer before and it was so hot out, and I remember kissing her and then thinking, 'Boy, this baby's sweat tastes salty.' But I had no idea. Why would I? So there we were . . . the lab guy finished getting Maggie set for the sweat test, and he told us to just walk around and come back in forty-five minutes or whatever it was. When we returned the poor guy was trembling. He had to tell us the diagnosis. 'Yes, Maggie has cystic fibrosis.' We went to see a specialist at Hinsdale Hospital the next day, and after the doctor talked to us for about fifteen minutes, Maggie was admitted to the hospital and we were inundated with, 'This is what she has. . . . This is how you do this. . . . This is what you're going to do. . . .' I just had no clue what was going on. I had a friend who had a friend who knew somebody. So she called. But it was one of those things where I didn't know if she was going to die today or in two weeks or what. I had no idea what to think. Someone went to the CF Foundation and got tons of information for me, and all I did was read and read the whole time Maggie was in the hospital. Everyone was so good to us and so nice. And Maggie seemed just fine. She was the hit of the hospital!

And then you just get used to it. It just becomes part of your life."

Nearly 89 percent of all funds raised by the Cystic Fibrosis Foundation are directed toward CF care, research, and education. In December 2003, the Wall Street Journal magazine *Smart Money* recognized the CF Foundation as the top charity in its health research category.

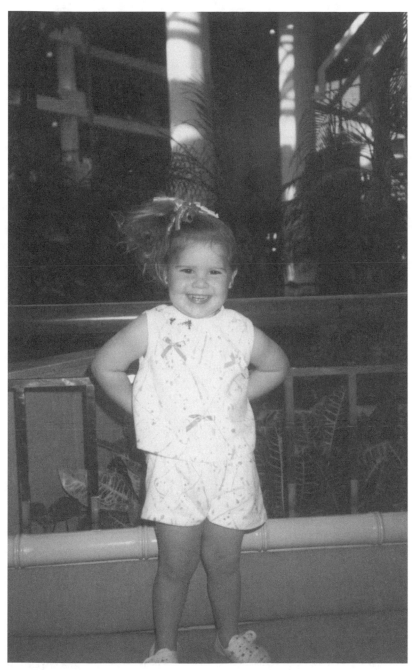

Maggie Sheehan at three years old, still the picture of health,
despite being diagnosed with CF two years earlier.

While statistically the majority of people who have cystic fibrosis are diagnosed before their third birthday, there is a small group of people for whom a diagnosis is not made until sometime later in life. In 1995 a seventy-two-year-old man from Portland, Oregon, was diagnosed with CF.[9]

A SURPRISE DIAGNOSIS DURING THE TEEN YEARS

While most CF diagnoses are made within the first two years of life, there are still a significant number of people who make it through childhood undiagnosed, only to have their symptoms flare to a point of obvious illness during adolescence. When this happens, the already tumultuous teen years can become a force to reckon with. After all, it's one thing to live all your life with an illness. You get used to it, in a sense. You know it's always been there and will always be there. It's another thing altogether to be going along as if you are as healthy as the next guy and then BAM! You're diagnosed with a serious, life-threatening illness. The kind of coping needed for this situation takes real strength.

"I am certain there are a lot of you out there who can't ever remember not being surrounded by cystic fibrosis, but I can. My children's diagnoses came late and both my kids were always healthy. It was very easy to be in denial about someone else's situations. I am not saying that I wasn't sympathetic to others' problems and illnesses, but they didn't really affect me, and when you don't live in it every day, people tend to forget what it really feels like and what you are really going through. My sister and her husband and family know what this disease is, and they know what we have been through. But they aren't in my house every day, listening to my kids coughing or vomiting or doing their treatments, so I think that they are able to tune it out for awhile. I know for a fact that I have become more sensitive since my kids were diagnosed—that I have even become overly sensitive, and I guess you could say even envious.

I work in a very small office with two other ladies who are in their 60s (I am in my 40s). It drives me over the edge when they hear about one of the elderly customers who has passed away. They say it's unfair and they don't understand, but when I talk about my kids, or they hear me on the phone with the doctors talking about their medical problems, they always compare them to someone they know who has asthma or allergies, or they tell me about the endless sore throats and coughs their kids had. I absolutely hate it, but I try and remember that their life has not been affected the way ours has—they just have no idea. I find that the less I talk to them about it, the better off I am.

I also feel that unless a disease is one that is quick moving and is visible, people don't think anything is wrong with your kids. If they were diagnosed with cancer, I believe people would be more understanding and sympathetic, maybe because they know what cancer is. People don't understand CF and they figure if it isn't affecting them immediately, then the kid must be okay, have gotten over it, or never had it in the first place. I sometimes want to bop them on the head and wake them up, but I don't think it would do any good. I figure that those are the same people who will eventually wake up and stand in complete shock

(*continued*)

43

with their hands in the air saying, "I never realized," when something does happen to your children. Then they will finally have to face what they didn't want to face in the first place.

Sometimes when people come into our office and they complain about their kids' tuition bills, I want to fly off the handle and tell them to get on bended knee and be thankful they have the opportunity to pay that bill. But then I realize that they really don't know what I am going through, and they really don't know that there are these kinds of situations out there. Sometimes it's very hard to stifle your thoughts and feelings. I realize that I might not see some things in life that others see with their kids, and that I might never have the chance to experience the fullness of their lives, but I also realize that I am the richest woman in the world for having such wonderful human beings as part of my life. They have taught me so much, and who'd have thought that teens could teach an old dog new tricks?

—Deborah Pence, Frankfort, Illinois, mom of teens Kevin and Olivia, both of whom have CF.

Olivia Pence, of Frankfort, Illinois, 17, talks about how she coped with finding out at age 12 that she had cystic fibrosis:

"I was 12 years old when I was diagnosed with cystic fibrosis. At the end of 1999, I had gotten the flu very badly. I didn't seem to recover at the rate that I should have been and I was still very sick in the beginning of 2000. I was very tired, fatigued, losing weight, lethargic, and I had on and off fever and night sweats. My mom continually took me back and forth to the pediatrician. The doctors took blood tests to see if they knew what was wrong with me. All the tests came back normal. They thought perhaps I had a problem with anorexia and made arrangements for us to see a nutritionist. My mom didn't believe it was anorexia and she insisted the doctors continue to test elsewhere. They thought that I had a bowel obstruction and even with X-rays on that, nothing showed up. Then I developed a slight cough and pain in the back under my lung so they tested for TB (tuberculosis). That was negative, too, but convinced that I had TB, they tested me again and tested my mom and brother, but again everyone was negative. They did a chest X-ray and saw spots in my lungs, and it was then that the doctor decided to admit me to the hospital, telling my mom he thought we might be dealing with lung cancer. My first hospitalization was May 25, 2000, and the final diagnosis was made on June 1, 2000. After I was admitted and had lots and lots of testing, including a sweat test, they diagnosed me with cystic fibrosis. We had never heard of the disease, and my mom had no clue that it ran genetically in the family. I have a brother who is now 19. He was diagnosed with CF at 15, not because he was sick but mainly because of the results of my sweat test.

"Even though my brother and I have the same gene mutation for this disease, we have totally different symptoms. I have a more severe case, and I suffer from lung damage, acid reflux, and anemia. I have had problems over the years with vomiting, and the doctors think that perhaps my pancreas is starting to fail. They will be doing an upper GI soon to see if it is that or an ulcer. My brother, on the other hand, has full lung capacity and no stomach problems, but he does have chronic sinusitis. He has had several sinus surgeries in the last couple of years. He had taken the diagnosis very hard emotionally, harder than me, even though I have a worse case of CF than he does.

"When my brother and I were first diagnosed, I think that it pulled us closer together. We would talk about it a lot and we would cry together. I think he felt that we shared a common bond. I feel, though, that over the years as my condition becomes worse, he has withdrawn from me. I think it is because he is afraid. I think that when he looks at me getting sicker, he sees his own mortality. But sometimes I feel that he doesn't care, and I feel that he is unable to help me when I am not feeling good. Although I really understand how he feels, or how he must feel, it still bothers me a little bit. I am worried about him. I guess with my brother being my only sibling, I am not sure how I would feel if I had a sibling *without* the same disease. I think my brother thinks differently than I do about the disease, and he worries more about his life and how long it will be, while I just live my life and believe that it will be a long, happy one.

"I usually wind up in the hospital once a year, not because of illness, but more on a 'tune-up' basis. I usually come home with a PICC (peripherally inserted central catheter) line for home IVs. This helps me come home a lot sooner.

"I am actually a sophomore in high school; however, I am still making up my missed work from freshman year. When I was in eighth grade, the school was very hard to deal with, with my disease, and it took them so long to get me a tutor that I just fell further and further behind when I would get sick. So, even though I was not at the same level with my classmates, my school still allowed me to graduate. I personally felt they wanted to rid themselves of my situation.

"I do chest physical therapy two times a day using the vest machine. I nebulize Pulmozyme once a day and Albuterol two times a day. I also take a daily dose of Nexium for my acid reflux. I am currently on Cipro for a slight infection. I don't currently participate in any sports, but I was involved in swimming before my diagnosis. I like to spend time with my friends, and I like chatting on the computer and talking on the phone. I think my health is better than most people with CF but that my disease has not progressed that far yet. When and if the time comes, I would consider a lung transplant but would be very afraid. I think that having CF has made me take a different look on life, and I don't take my life for granted. The worst thing about having CF is being sick lots of the time and not doing what I would like to do. The biggest challenge to me as a teenager with CF is that other teenagers who don't have the disease just don't understand, no matter how hard they try. They can never understand. My friends know I have CF. My boyfriend and I were talking about running one day, and I told him I would not be able to run for a far distance. He asked me

Did You Know?
Pop singer Celine Dion's niece Karine died from cystic fibrosis in 1993 at age 16. Celine's song "Fly," which appears as the final track on her CD *Falling Into You*, was written in Karine's memory. Celine has been promoting CF awareness since 1982, and in 1993 she became the National Celebrity Patron of the CF Foundation.

why not, and I told him about my disease. His response to this was, 'What is that?' Once I had told him what it was he wanted to find out more about it. He is very understanding about it.

"I have lots of plans for the future. I don't plan on going to college. For my career I would like to become a hairdresser. As for marriage, yes, I plan on getting married and having kids. I currently do not have CF-related diabetes and personally pray it never happens; I am a chocolate addict and don't think I could survive without my daily fix of chocolate!

Today a person living in the United States who has CF can expect to live to a median age of 35.1 years. A person who had CF back in 1986 could only expect to see his or her 15th birthday.

"If I could tell other teens one thing about CF, it's this: Just because doctors say you have so long to live, or the median life span is 30 years old, he or she has no idea when someone is going to die. I think that you should live life to the fullest and have plans for the future!"

ADULT DIAGNOSIS

Of course, the truly late diagnosis, the one that comes in adulthood, presents perhaps the most outrageous of challenges, as it often requires an almost complete lifestyle change. Coping with this can be a monumental task. Henry*, a 34-year-old man from Kansas, shares his intimate story of how he was diagnosed with cystic fibrosis at age 32.

"My wife and I couldn't conceive a baby, so we went to a fertility specialist. He diagnosed me with absence of the vas deferens, which is common in males with cystic fibrosis. He suggested I be tested for CF. Several months later I had the sweat test and genetic test that confirmed that I do have cystic fibrosis. No one else in my family has CF that I know of. It was hard finding out that I couldn't have children and that I might not live a long life.

"Since my diagnosis two years ago, I had to go on disability and give up my job. I had worked for almost twenty years, but it became too physical and difficult for me. It is very hard not to work and earn a living. The hardest part for me is not being able to financially take care of my family (my wife and three dogs). I have to rely on Social Security Disability, which doesn't pay much. My wife works. It was also hard to get used to going to the doctor so often and taking so much medication.

"I have a fairly mild case of CF, but I have severe lung damage due to the many years of not being treated. However, it is hard to make a prognosis because anything could happen. I just try to stay as healthy as possible and take care of myself. Since most people are diagnosed at a young age, they grow up knowing about their CF, learning how to take care of themselves. They get used to the doctors and hospital visits and treatments, and it just all becomes a part of their lives and who they are. It allows them the opportunity to plan for their future by going to college or choosing a field that they can physically handle for a longer period of time. They are able to tell their mate before marriage. Their family knows about it and learns about it and, in most cases, are there for them. I never had these advantages. It was all thrown at me at age 32. My whole life changed in an instant. My wife's life changed as well. It is very different being diagnosed in adulthood versus in childhood, at least in my opinion.

"I think more people need to know that adults can be diagnosed with cystic fibrosis. My CF nurse told me they always considered any diagnosis after six years of age to be a late diagnosis! They've had a few cases of adult diagnosis in the last few years. She said it is hard for people diagnosed later to adjust and cope with it. Imagine my shock at age 32! I am still learning to cope. It is a day-to-day process. It is a shame that so many people still die so young. Sometimes I wonder why I am different. Don't get me wrong, I am definitely glad to be here. I hope I am here for many more years, and I hope I'm here to see the cure, even if it is too late for me to benefit from it."

ANOTHER BOOK WORTH READING

Jacquie Gordon writes about the life of her daughter, Christine, who has cystic fibrosis, in *Give Me One Wish* (New York: W. W. Norton & Co. Inc., 1988). Christine wants more than anything to live life as a normal teenager, to go to high school and college, to perform in theatrical productions, and to fall in love. Christine lives life to the fullest, thanks in part to her mother's understanding that, for Christine, she has just a few years to live a lifetime of experiences.

NOTES

1. CysticFibrosis.com, www.cysticfibrosis.com/info/symptoms.html.

2. Arizona Respiratory Center, www.resp-sci.arizona.edu/patient-info/child/cystic-fibrosis-k.htm.

3. Cincinnati Children's Hospital Medical Center, www.cincinattichildrens.org/health/info/chest/diagnose/cf-diagnosis.htm.

4. University of Wisconsin Medical School, Department of Pediatrics, "Sweat Testing," www.pediatrics.wisc.edu/childrenshosp/sweat/sweat.html.

5. "Sweat Testing."

6. Cystic Fibrosis Trust, www.cftrust.org.uk/meeting_point/faqs_adults.htm.

7. Cystic Fibrosis Trust.

8. Cincinnati Children's Hospital Medical Center, www.cincinattichildrens.org/health/info/chest/diagnose/cf-diagnosis.htm.

9. Norma Kennedy Plourde's Cystic Fibrosis website, personal.nbnet.nb.ca/nnormap/CF.htm, or www3.nbnet.nb.ca/normap/cfhistory.htm.

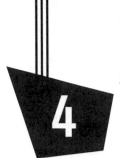

A Daily Challenge

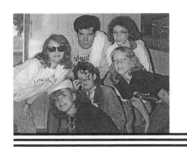

If we were lucky, our alarm clocks would go off, and we'd awaken to that annoying but steady and familiar "beep, beep, beep." If we were unlucky, someone—usually one of the overzealous nurses—would come along with a bullhorn. From cabin door to cabin door she'd blast us with something like, "Wake up! Fifteen minutes until therapy!" Bleary-eyed and shivering in the chill of the early August morning, campers trudged through grass still wet with dew, to a large cabin that bore the ironic name "Fun Lodge." There, as the sun rose around us and warmed the air back to summer temperatures, campers, therapists, nurses, and I partook in the first of two daily therapy sessions, which helped the campers breathe more easily so as to enjoy the activities of the day.

"A child with cystic fibrosis never merely lives. She must be kept alive."
—Frank Deford, from his book *Alex: The Life of a Child*.[1]

While there remains no cure for cystic fibrosis, the therapies recommended for people who have cystic fibrosis have undergone radical changes in the past twenty or so years. Frank Deford, in his poignant 1983 memoir of the short life of his daughter Alex, writes about Alex's nights sleeping under a dewy, cloudy mist tent. Meant to moisten secretions in the lungs throughout the night, the tents, which enclosed both the child and his or her bed, were often thought to do more psychological damage than physical good. Today, the same moistening of secretions is accomplished in a much simpler manner via a machine called the nebulizer.

THE NEBULIZER

"To loosen mucus I nebulize with saltwater, which I just mix on my own," says Alice Vosloo, 19, of Port Elizabeth, South Africa. While there are a number of different types of nebulizers—or "nebs" as they are usually called by those who use them frequently—the basics of how to use a common nebulizer (the kind most people who have CF use at home) are simple. A prescribed amount of medication—or as Alice Vosloo described, saline (or saltwater)—is placed into a small cup. The cup is attached at one end, via a length of plastic tubing, to a small machine, the nebulizer, which generally requires a source of electricity for power. The other, wider, end of the cup is attached to a wider piece of plastic tubing, one end of which holds a mouthpiece or a facemask (which covers the mouth and nose). When the nebulizer is turned on, air flows through the thinner tubing and turns the liquid medication into an aerosol, which can be breathed into the lungs. An aerosol looks like steam or smoke but is actually the medication, which has been reduced to tiny particle size, small enough to be inhaled and to reach both the larger and smaller airways of the lungs. The aerosol is breathed in through the mouthpiece (or facemask) using slow, steady breaths. "An end-inspiratory hold facilitates deposition."[2] This means that taking a deep breath and holding it helps the medication reach all parts of the lungs.

For small children or anyone who might feel too sick or too weak to hold the mouthpiece, a facemask, which covers the mouth and nose, can be used. Very small babies are often given their nebulizer medications using a method called blow-by, or flow-by, in which the mouthpiece is removed from the larger bit of tubing and that end sealed off (usually with a bit of surgical tape) and the medication is allowed to simply blow out the other end and into the general direction of the baby's mouth and nose.

Unfortunately, even with the most coordinated breathing, only about 8 to 12 percent of an aerosolized medication actually reaches the lungs of an adult. In children the percentage is even less. The majority of the medication is lost in the atmosphere. This is why, for the

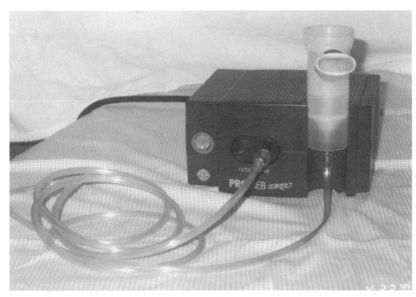

Nebulizer

best possible outcome, it is so important to follow the prescribed method of deep breaths and breath holds and to finish all of the medication in the cup each time.

Most people who have cystic fibrosis begin and end their day with nebulizer treatments.

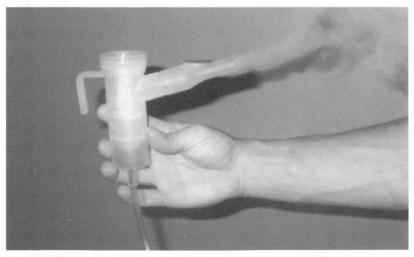

The smokelike mist blowing out of the PARI neb's mouthpiece is medication normally inhaled through the mouth and into the lungs.

Albuterol, also known as Ventolin and Proventil, is one of the most common medications used by people who have respiratory problems (not only cystic fibrosis but also asthma, for example). Albuterol is a bronchodilator, which means it opens the airways to make breathing easier and to allow the mucus a chance to escape. Xopenex, a newer drug that came out in recent years, works much the same way that Albuterol

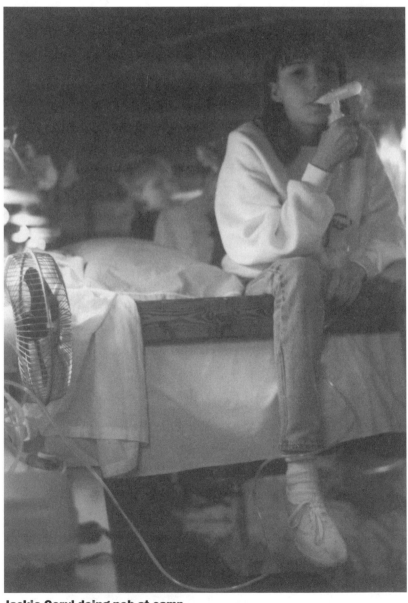

Jackie Goryl doing neb at camp

works but without the common side effects of Albuterol, such as shaky hands, nervousness, and increased heart rate.

Other medications can be nebulized and aerosolized, as well. One of the most

> **"Every morning I wake up and do my Albuterol neb. This is probably the most important med [medicine] for the day because if I don't do it, I will be wheezy and short of breath for the entire day," says Jackie Goryl, 23.**

popular drugs to hit the CF circuit in the 1990s is called Pulmozyme®, Dornase, or most commonly, DNAse. DNAse, which was approved by the FDA in 1993, is a genetically engineered form of the human enzyme deoxyribonuclease. DNAse works by breaking up the human genetic material called deoxyribonucleic acid, the "junk" DNA found in large quantities in the lungs' secretions. By breaking down the DNA, it reduces the thickness of the secretions to unplug the airways and reduce the opportunity for infections in the lungs. It is usually inhaled during Vest therapy or following manual bronchial drainage (both of which you will soon read about).[3]

Once the mucus in the lungs has been loosened and coughed out, the cleaner lungs are often given a dose of antibiotics. Inhaled antibiotics work to kill off bacteria living in the lungs and to prevent new bacteria from growing and causing infection. In recent years several new antibiotics have become available to fight chronic lung infections. One of the latest drugs is azithromycin, which is an antibiotic that has recently proven to be effective in people with cystic fibrosis whose lungs are chronically infected with the common *Pseudomonas aeruginosa* bacteria.[4]

"I take the Colistin inhaled treatment every other month," says Jessica Hawk-Manus. A fairly new antibiotic, Colistin is prescribed in a one-month-on, one-month-off fashion. Another new medication that came out in the late 1990s is called TOBI®. At one time, Tobramycin, a commonly prescribed intravenous (IV) antibiotic, was mixed with saline and inhaled. TOBI® is a form of Tobramycin that was created specifically for inhalation. The advantage to the inhaled form is that it reaches the infected lung tissue directly, which in turn reduces the amount of the drug necessary to fight the infection. It reduces the likelihood of possible side effects, as well.

Older people who have cystic fibrosis might recall taking medications with names like viokase (an enzyme), mucomyst (which many might remember as the medicine that "smelled like rotten eggs" and has been essentially replaced by the newer drug, DNAse), bronkosol, and alupent. Today these are not well known or widely used by the CF population.

IS THE ORDER IMPORTANT?

Often these questions come up: Does it matter in what order I do my nebulizer treatments? Can I mix two or more medications in my nebulizer to save time? The answer to the first question is: Yes! The answer to the second is: No!

Follow these guidelines when doing your nebulizer treatments because the order in which you do your nebs is *very* important. Their effectiveness relies on it.

1. Bronchodilator (such as Albuterol or Xopenex) **FIRST** to open up your lungs (*before* manual chest therapy or *during* Vest)
2. Mucolytic (DNAse) **SECOND** to help break up the mucus and allow you to cough it out (*after* manual chest therapy or *during* Vest)
3. Antibiotic (TOBI®, Colistin, etc.) **LAST** so as to allow it to reach the cleanest lung tissue possible (*after* manual chest therapy or Vest and *after* coughing and clearing of the lungs)

Think about what would happen if you inhaled your antibiotic before coughing and clearing your lungs. You would simply be allowing the antibiotic to settle on the mucus, and then you'd lose it all when you coughed the mucus out. It's very important to follow the three steps and do your nebs in this order. For obvious reasons, then, it would not be productive to mix your medications to "save time." There are also problems with some of the medications reacting poorly with one another within the nebulizer cup itself and causing the equipment to clog. When in doubt, check with your respiratory therapist or, better yet, check with the drug company that manufactures your medication in question.

> **"The first nebulizer I took as a kid was Gentamycin."**
> **—Mike L., Baltimore, Maryland**

MORE MEDS: THE MDI

If you know anyone who has asthma you have undoubtedly seen him or her whip out an MDI and take a puff now and then. The MDI, or metered dose inhaler, has come to be commonly used by people who have CF as well. A whole list of medications, from Albuterol, which opens the airways, to various inhaled steroids, which reduce swelling, can now be taken by MDI. While easy to use and certainly less time consuming than a ten- to fifteen-minute nebulizer treatment, there is uncertainty regarding whether or not some medications, such as Albuterol, are more effective in nebulized form. Nonetheless, many people with CF use one or more MDIs as part of their daily treatment regimen. Most MDIs use a standard two-puff dose, each of which is taken with a deep breath followed by a hold, followed by a thirty- to sixty-second wait to allow the medication to reach down into the lungs, and then a repeat of this process with the second puff. To be done properly, an MDI should be used with a spacer or aerochamber, which is a plastic mouthpiece device that helps the medication to be breathed into the lungs rather than deposited in the mouth. For babies and small children, a spacer with a mask attached is used, and the child is required to take six breaths to completely inhale the full dose of the medication. When used without the spacer, the MDI delivers very little medication to the lungs and is therefore rather ineffective. It is possible to learn a proper technique of taking an MDI without the spacer, but it takes a great deal of concentration and coordination.

IVs AND ORAL MEDICATIONS

As you might have already figured out, one of the staples of treatment for those who have cystic fibrosis is medication, not only inhaled but also IV and oral. The exact regimen of daily oral medications will vary from person to person, with some people taking little more than enzymes and vitamins and others practically making a meal out of their many pills. Those who have cystic fibrosis learn to take their pills at a young age, and they learn to take many at a time. It has been claimed that five pills is "no sweat for someone who has CF" and even ten pills swallowed at once is not uncommon. Faela Smyth, 16, of Dublin, Ireland, quips, "I decided one time I would truly discover quite how many tablets I could take at once. It's really remarkable the things we CFers get up to on a daily basis. Well, I got it up to eighteen and, boy, am I proud!" To give you an idea what someone who has CF might take on a daily basis, Chad Lucci, 26, suggests one might take steroids to reduce inflammation in the lungs; prophylactic antibiotics; various GI (gastrointestinal) meds for problems such as acid reflux and other CF-related issues; a multivitamin; and of course enzymes with snacks and meals. Chad also remembers taking salt replacement tablets as a child. "They were big horse pills," Chad recalls.

It takes a lot of work to fight cystic fibrosis. And sometimes all these pills don't do enough and one is said to have a CF exacerbation. When someone is suffering from an exacerbation, he or she might then consider him- or herself sick. The infection in his or her lungs gets to be too much for oral antibiotics alone and IV medications become necessary. The advantage of the IV over the oral medications is that they go directly into the bloodstream. And in the case of the PICC line, the antibiotics can go right to the valves of the heart and can be pumped better for rapid circulation though the body. Until recently the need for IV antibiotics also meant the need for hospitalization. Now, thanks to technology and visiting nurses, many people who have CF are able to complete a round of antibiotics in the comfort of their own home. A trip to the hospital is still necessary for the insertion of the IV or the PICC line, but the course of the medication can be given at home.

Over the years, much of the improvement in the prognosis of CF can be attributed to the ongoing research that continues to yield new and better medications. Recently a new drug has been approved to fight *Pseudomonas*. Ciprofloxacin, an antibiotic that is taken orally could, for some, act as effectively as a course of intravenous antibiotics.[5]

Ibuprofen, the anti-inflammatory component of many over-the-counter painkillers, such as Motrin® and Advil®, was tested and found to reduce inflammation in the lungs. This, in turn, curbs the damage and helps maintain lung function, as well as body weight. In the trial for the drug, people who had CF were given high doses of ibuprofen twice a day for four years. The treatment was found to work best and have the best result on kids under 13 years old. It is important to note that ibuprofen therapy might not be for everyone as the drug itself carries some potential side effects that might outweigh the benefits. While ibuprofen is easy to get because it is an over-the-counter medicine, it is very important to discuss this drug therapy with a doctor before trying it.[6]

CHEST PHYSICAL THERAPY BY ANY OTHER NAME . . .

One of the hallmark treatments for cystic fibrosis is airway clearance. While the chronic cough itself works to clear the airways of mucus, it is not enough to reach the hard-to-evacuate nooks and crannies of the lungs. Over the years, methods of therapy to clear the airways have been improved upon time and again. Yet for some, the gold standard, manual chest physical therapy performed by a dedicated caregiver (usually a parent, respiratory therapist, or nurse) is still the favorite. If you talk to five different people who have CF you will learn five different names for this therapy that is applied directly to the walls of the chest in order to physically loosen the mucus inside. Pounding, clapping, BD (short for bronchial drainage), PD (short for postural drainage), cupping, thumping, CPT (short for chest physical therapy), pats, tapping, physiotherapy, exercises, and therapy—all of these names mean the exact same treatment. For our purposes, we'll rely on chest therapy as our term of favor.

Properly done chest therapy consists of pounding on each lobe of the lungs with cupped hands while the person who has CF sits up straight, lies flat on his back, lies flat on his stomach, and lies on each side. Then he or she will lie in each of these positions again but with his or her head lower than his or her feet to allow gravity to assist, and pounding in all positions (except sitting straight up) will be repeated. Each section will optimally be pounded on for at least five minutes and a full treatment will take roughly thirty to forty-five minutes. This is "optimal" but not necessarily "actual." For most, a therapy session might take about twenty minutes or so. Coupled with the nebulizer medications taken before and after the chest therapy, a full session of therapy should take well over an hour.

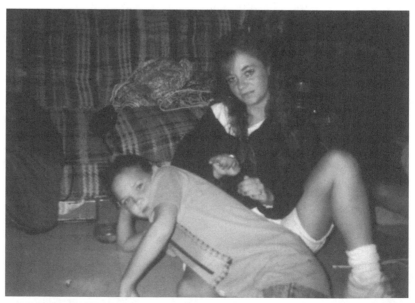

Here I am giving Candice Budnieski her chest therapy at CF camp in the early 1990s.

And because it is difficult to reach all areas of the chest on oneself, chest therapy is generally performed by another person, usually a parent, older sibling, or other caregiver.

Chest therapy has been called "primitive" by many. And in truth, it is. Think about it. Someone is banging on your chest to whack out the mucus to make it easier for you to cough it out. Thump, thump, thump! When done properly, this sometimes uncomfortable, though not intentionally painful, treatment can be heard echoing down the halls of a hospital or throughout the house. It definitely warrants turning up the volume on the television. Perhaps the biggest challenge to chest therapy, aside from finding the time to do it properly and effectively, is getting small children to stay still long enough to get it done. Mike DiBiase talked about his childhood experience with chest therapy in a 1996 interview. "We didn't even get therapy at home. We didn't even do it," Mike said, describing how relatively normal the early years were for him and his younger sister Jenny. "I remember once when my parents got the diagrams on how to do the treatments. Then they did it for a while. Perhaps they should have been stricter with it. Jenny and I were not really cooperative with our treatments. We wouldn't want to sit down and get pounded. We were out[side], too busy running around playing."

Another great challenge to traditional chest physical therapy is the need for someone to perform the treatment. It is relatively simple to pound your own front and sides, but giving yourself a good, effective treatment is not easy to accomplish. Luckily for Mike and Jenny and others like them, those who described the chest therapy as "primitive" were also looking toward the future for those who

> **"The big difference between CF therapies of the past and today is not the drugs as much as the choices in airway clearance techniques that we never had before,"** says Joanne Salazar, who works in the Pulmonary Function Testing (PFT) Lab at Children's Memorial Hospital in Chicago.

have CF. They were looking at the fact that many are now living longer and on into adulthood. There was a growing need for an independent method of providing chest therapy.

THE VEST

"I use the Vest twice a day with ten minutes at 10Hz (pressure 5.5, full vest) and then ten minutes at 15Hz (5.5 pressure)," James Lawlor, 17, says, describing his twice daily regimen with the greatest technological advance since, well, perhaps since the decision to take down those mist tents.

Created by a company called American Biosystems, the Vest™, which was originally called the ThAIRapy Vest, provides airway clearance by way of an actual vest worn by the person with CF:

> The main components of the Vest include the air-pulse generator and an inflatable vest. The generator is electrically powered and consists of a two-stage vacuum blower and a motor driven bellows. The inflatable vest is made from vinyl material and has two ports located on the front. Large bore tubing connects the vest to the air-pulse generator. The purpose of the Vest is to provide airway clearance through mechanical high frequency chest wall oscillation (HFCWO). It works by creating pulses of air, which cause the vest to inflate and then deflate against the thorax. By constricting the thorax, the inflatable vest causes a decrease in end expiratory lung volume (EELV).[7]

Or, in the words of 18-year-old James Lawlor, daily Vest user:

> "The Vest has two main settings: pressure and hertz, (Hz, cycles per second). The pressure indicates how much the Vest inflates and is mainly a comfort issue. The Hz is the frequency of the pulses delivered by the Vest. I remember hearing that different frequencies work on different sections of the lungs. I really couldn't tell you what the significance is of my particular regimen (ten minutes at 10Hz and ten minutes at 15Hz), other than it's what my doctor prescribed. There's really no one 'standard' that Vest users use. As for the term *full vest*, the Vest now has two different actual vests that you can get: the full vest, which goes all the way down to the waist and inflates all

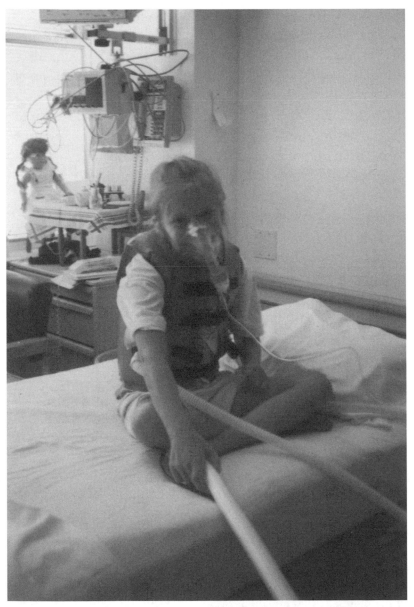

During this 1995 hospital stay Katie Kocelko receives her nebulized medications via a facemask nebulizer, while using the Vest.

around, and the chest vest, which only extends to the top of the abdomen and doesn't inflate quite as much but is just as effective. I ended up getting the full vest and it works for me, although someone I know says the full vest makes his stomach hurt when he uses it or when he's having a bad GI (gastrointestinal) day."

A Vest treatment takes about thirty minutes. "Depending on my mood or what I am doing during therapy, I sometimes leave the Vest on the whole time I do the nebs. If I am playing video games, sometimes I don't pay attention to the timer and end up doing therapy for hours," says Janelle Benitez*. While traditional chest therapy can only target one specific area of the lungs at a time, the Vest reaches all areas of the lungs throughout the entire session of therapy. According to American Biosystems, this is one of the reasons why the Vest has been reported to be three times more effective than manual chest physical therapy in mobilizing secretions.[8] The other advantages to the Vest versus traditional chest therapy are that it can be done independently and that the nebulizer can be used at the same time as the Vest because the person using it sits upright throughout the treatment. While the machine that powers the actual Vest is large and somewhat cumbersome, and the cost of the contraption is roughly the same as that of a small car (most insurance plans cover the cost of its use), the benefits definitely outweigh these minor inconveniences. Because of the Vest, teens have been able to go off to college with a great tool for airway clearance, whereas once they would have been confined to attempts to perform chest therapy on themselves, recruit a dormmate to help out, or simply forgo either the chest therapy or college altogether. Young adults find living alone, independently, to be much easier for the same reasons.

For more information on how the Vest is specifically used, visit classes.kumc.edu/cahe/respcared/cybercas/cysticfibrosis/tracpurp.html or contact the company that makes the Vest, American Biosystems, Inc., 20 Yorktown Court, St. Paul, Minnesota 55117 (phone: 651-415-9316, fax: 651-490-1484, e-mail: ltoskey@abivest.com).

In addition to the Vest, which has been approved for children as young as two years old, other smaller devices have been created to aid in the clearance of the airways.

PEP, FLUTTER, AND ACAPELLA

Since the early 1990s, three small, handheld devices have become available to people who have cystic fibrosis. The first handheld device is the PEP. Working on the principle of positive expiratory pressure, PEP therapy is done by blowing into a small plastic device that provides resistance to the airways, much in the way blowing through the small diameter of a drinking straw would. The PEP device can be hooked up to a nebulizer and both the airway clearance and the medications are delivered at the same time.

Following the PEP device, the Flutter came along. The Flutter is similar to PEP in that it employs a small, plastic, handheld device. Blowing into the Flutter, however, activates a small ball bearing to bounce—or flutter—quickly up and down, creating a vibration that travels into the lungs.

Acapella is a larger and newer, handheld device that combines the positive expiratory pressure of the PEP device and the vibration of the Flutter while also delivering the aerosolized medications.

"The advantage of Acapella over Flutter is that Acapella is a little easier to use. It is not as easily affected by the position in which it is held. Also, it is possible to use it in conjunction with a nebulizer. You can actually do the

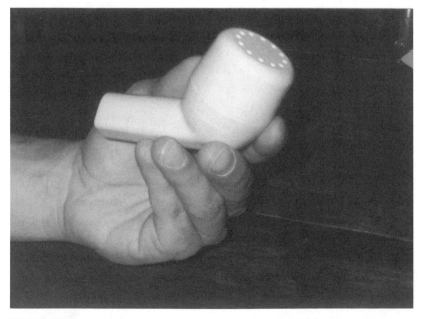

The Flutter

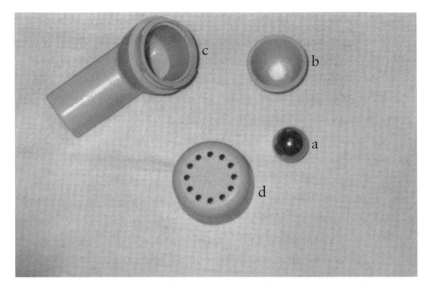

The Flutter taken apart to show its inner components. The metal ball (a) sits in the cup (b), which sits in the device itself (c). The cap (d), which has holes in it for exhaled air to escape, is screwed onto part c. The metal ball actually flutters up and down during exhalation, causing a vibration in the lungs.

Acapella and the neb simultaneously, and it can be used with any of the medications. Since it is PEP and vibration all at once, it actually serves a twofold purpose. During the neb treatment, the positive expiratory pressure (PEP) helps to 'stint' the airways open, and many people feel that this enhances medication delivery to the airways. It's also good to use after treatments (especially after DNAse) because the vibrations help break loose the thinned secretions."—Mike Shoemaker, respiratory therapist, Easley, South Carolina

Which device one chooses is merely a matter of preference. The PEP and Flutter devices can be easily stored in a purse or bookbag, while the Acapella requires a bit more traveling room.

ANYTHING ELSE?

Some very coordinated, diligent, and self-motivated people have successfully learned to perform autogenic drainage. Unlike the other forms of airway clearance, which require some sort of device or at the very least another pair of hands, autogenic drainage is done with a combination of mental concentration and physical coordination. Using a technique composed of a series of various levels of breathing, autogenic drainage moves secretions up the lungs until they are ready to be coughed out using a technique called the "huff." A "huff" cough is done by taking a deep breath and then expelling the breath slowly but forcefully through the mouth. The first level of breathing used in autogenic drainage is a low-lung volume breathing that loosens the mucus. Then, using a midvolume breathing, mucus is "collected." The final stage is the "huff" cough to clear the mucus from the lungs.

If this all sounds complicated, the truth of the matter is, it is. But this is not to say that it cannot be learned with a little bit (ok, a lot!) of discipline, concentration, and coaching. Those who have learned to do autogenic drainage properly will realize the many advantages, such as not having to drag equipment along, not having to rely on others for help, and having everything necessary to ensure an effective method of airway clearance wherever they go. In addition, autogenic drainage is a gentler method of airway clearance than some of the other more popular methods. This can be especially helpful if you are prone to bouts of hemoptysis (coughing up blood).

TAKE YOUR PICK

There is no right, or best, method of airway clearance. You will undoubtedly have a personal preference as to what works best for you in clearing your lungs of mucus. When asked, a group of people who have CF and the parents of children who have CF gave testimony that the methods they use work well. Some swear by the Vest, others prefer the mobility of the smaller handheld devices, and still others prefer the "good old-fashioned" manual chest therapy. Some people prefer one method for a while and then switch to something different for various reasons. There are even some people who choose to exercise vigorously rather than partake in a more traditional form of airway clearance. However, before making this decision for yourself, it is important to consult your CF doctor.

Jackie Goryl uses both the Flutter and the Vest, depending on how much time she has and how she feels on any given day:

"As far as physiotherapy, I am not the most compliant. I have the Vest and a Flutter. I like the Vest, as I feel it does a better job, but it is time consuming (thirty minutes twice a day). That is especially difficult to fit in during school, but I try my best. When I am sicker, I make sure to do some method of physiotherapy as it will help me get better quicker."

☺

"I definitely do Flutter every night. That's one thing I'm very consistent with because I actually feel as if this helps me."—Jennifer Cherry

☺

"I start my day at 7:30 a.m. I do a thirty- to forty-five-minute treatment then rush to get ready to leave on the 8:40 school bus. I do a Serevent (a bronchodilator) MDI, then I start the Vest. While I'm on the Vest I do my DNAse, and when the Vest is done I do the TOBI®. I only take the Albuterol when I am in the hospital. It takes too much time and so I don't do it at home."—Maggie Sheehan, 15

☺

"She still did her nebs every day plus she was doing her Vest a little bit, but mainly I did her therapy. And if she had given up, I knew she wouldn't have been doing those things. And she did them every day, religiously."—Mike DiBiase, on therapy during his sister Jenny's final months

It's important to find a method of airway clearance that is most helpful to you and a routine that you are not only comfortable with but that also leaves you breathing more comfortably and prepared to go about your day.

"My daily regimen goes like this: I take five or six Ultrase MT20 enzyme capsules with meals and three to five with snacks. I take Zantac (an antiulcer drug) 150 mg twice a day and ADEKS (multivitamin) twice a day. I use the Vest twice a day with ten minutes at 10Hz (pressure 5.5, full vest) and then ten minutes at 15Hz (5.5 pressure). I would like to get started on a regimen of Zithromax (an antibiotic) for inflammation control and mucus thinning, so I plan to ask my doctor about that again at our next appointment (in the next month or so). I also try to exercise every day on our exercise machine. Right now I'm working up to a thirty-minute aerobic workout every day (usually around two miles at this point) and then an additional twelve-minute strength training/muscle toning workout Monday, Wednesday, and Friday."—James Lawlor, 17

Alice Vosloo describes her daily regimen:

"I nebulize with saltwater to loosen mucus or Pulmozyme® (our medical aid only allows us about four boxes a year) once or twice a day, depending on how my chest feels. I'm also supposed to do postural drainage twice a day for ten minutes. I also take about eight to ten Creon 10000 capsules a day with meals. Then there's obviously also multivitamins and oral antibiotics when needed (which is most of the time)."

Janelle Benitez's routine is planned down to every detail:

"I get up in the morning and do an hour of therapy or breathing treatment. I spend about a half hour in my Vest and do Albuterol nebs at the same time. After the Albuterol is gone, I do TOBI® or Colistin depending on which one I am on at the time. (I alternate them each month.) Then I shower and get ready. Before I brush my teeth I do Advair (an MDI). I find keeping it with my toothbrush is convenient because it reminds me to do it, and I know I am not going to get thrush from it if I am brushing right afterwards.

"At night before bed I do the Vest again with the Albuterol, my DNAse, and the TOBI® or Colistin. Then I wash my face, do my Advair again, and gargle with Listerine for a count of sixty. I take all my meds at night because I find the vitamins don't upset my stomach then, and my antacid is supposed to be taken at night. Since none of my meds are required to be in the morning, it just made sense to save time and do them all at once at night. Plus, I was getting sick to my stomach in the morning from my vitamins, so it made sense to try to switch them. I find that keeping the meds next to my bed on the nightstand is also convenient. I just take a glass of water to bed with me and take the meds. Having them right there out in the open is just another good way to remind myself because I see them. Plus, if I am feeling lazy there are no excuses because they're right there."

BREATHE IN, BREATHE OUT

Sometimes the biggest challenge of the day is much simpler than trying to fit in or trying to make time for therapy. Sometimes just breathing itself presents the greatest challenge of all.

"Every night at camp I listened to my cabinmates cough while we should have been sleeping. At first I wondered if I should go get someone to help, but I soon came to realize that this kind of coughing was not unusual and as soon as a spasm would pass, maybe after five minutes, or maybe after ten, we'd all just go back to sleep. No one ever bothered to call out, 'Are you ok?' in the dark of our cabin. She, whichever girl was coughing, could not have replied anyway. The cough usually began with a few short bursts, perhaps some throat clearing. When it became apparent to the cougher that more coughing was about to come, she would take as deep a breath as possible, for she knew it would be a frighteningly long while before she would be able to catch her breath again. The mucus would seem to literally roll inside her chest as one cough led into another with no audible breath or even a chance to spit out this vile stuff in between. She would shake from the effort and her face would become a deep shade of red. And I would wonder how, with all that mucus inside her, could she breathe at all?"—Melanie Ann Apel

COUGH, COUGH, COUGH

The hallmark sign of cystic fibrosis is the cough. At times the cough is specific and deliberate, such as during a therapy session. After all the nebulizers and pounding, the lungs are open and the mucus is loose and it is prime time to get to work coughing out as much of the mucus—"yucky," "secretions," "samples," "gloopy glob" (Laura Tillman), "stinky-monas" (for the odor associated with

pseudomonas)—as possible. Half a box of tissues later the lungs are fairly clear. A couple hours of easy breathing should follow, with relatively little coughing.

Often just mildly interruptive, a cough might come here or there in short bursts. But for those who are in more advanced stages of the disease, coughing becomes a much bigger part of the day. Sounding loose and rattly, similar to that of a smoker, the cough of cystic fibrosis is deep and powerful—and unmistakable.

It's no wonder, then, that quite often vomiting follows a bout of coughing.

NUTRITION AND EXERCISE

In addition to the challenges young people face trying to fit twice-daily therapy into their already busy routine, many teens admit that maintaining a proper diet and getting regular exercise can become challenges as well.

When it comes to the importance of diet and exercise, CF allows no exceptions. Because of the body's inability to break down fats and properly digest foods without the properly functioning pancreas and its pancreatic enzymes, doctors originally prescribed low-fat diets for their CF patients. That meant no chocolate, no french fries, no fried chicken or pizza, no frosting or cake. Imagine a childhood without the fun foods that usually go hand in hand with birthday parties! Such a diet was meant to keep digestive problems to a minimum. Of course, if your body's digestive system is impaired because of pancreatic insufficiency, the result is that regardless of what you eat, no food—fatty or otherwise—will stay with you for long.

Today, doctors recognize the need for proper nutrition much better than they did years ago. In the days before cystic fibrosis even had a name, and even in the years after cystic fibrosis was officially "discovered," nutritional problems played as big a role in children's ultimate deaths as did the respiratory component of CF.

Now, most people who have cystic fibrosis take replacement enzymes, which allow them to absorb the nutrients in their food almost as well as those who don't have CF. (It is interesting to note here that not all people who have CF suffer from the pancreatic insufficiency, and therefore not all people who have CF require enzyme pills.) However, the enzyme pills are not a cure for the problem, and some people who have cystic fibrosis are still smaller in stature and weight than they might have been if they had not had CF (based on the relative size of other family members, especially their parents and healthy siblings). It might seem that taking more enzymes in an attempt to correct the problem would help, but in fact the opposite is true: taking more enzymes can actually cause more problems. High doses of pancreatic enzyme supplements have been associated with the development of colonic strictures (a narrowing of the colon), also known as fibrosing colonopathy. CF doctors are now more cautious when prescribing doses of the enzymes.[9]

What has been found to work better for people with CF is a balanced diet with more attention paid to calories. While kids with CF were once steered away from foods high in fat and calories, now they are encouraged to take in as many calories as they can reasonably eat. Compromised lungs require a great deal of extra energy to work. Energy comes to the body in the form of calories. So, choosing wisely among high-nutrition foods, those who have CF can pretty much eat up! Vitamin supplements are also helpful in maintaining proper nutrition. It has also been found that those who are able to maintain adequate nutritional status, along with a regular exercise program, have a better chance of fighting off bacterial infections.

WHO WANTS TO EAT?

In addition to the cough, another other classic symptom of cystic fibrosis is the appetite. Small children who have not yet been diagnosed with cystic fibrosis will eat and eat yet remain tiny, often losing weight rather than gaining. Once CF is diagnosed, enzyme supplements are prescribed and food is digested properly. Yet many who have CF still remain on the thin side. Why do you suppose that is?

When a healthy person gets an ordinary cold his or her nose becomes stuffed up, and it's hard to breathe without opening his or her mouth. Eating is difficult because it's nearly impossible to breathe through the mouth and chew at the same time. Many kids and young adults who have CF describe their everyday feeling as "a bad chest cold." So it's no wonder eating is not a favorite event. Another reason why it's not much fun to eat when you have CF is that coughing, especially after a meal, often results in the partial or total loss of lunch! More serious is the need for control. Especially in the younger teens, eating often becomes a struggle for control. "They can make me take pills, do therapy, nebs," says Cary*, "but they can't make me eat." Yet another reason for not eating is simply the lack of interest and energy to eat. And when everyone is always telling you, "eat, eat," it's just no fun anymore.

WHEN ALL ELSE FAILS: SUPPLEMENTAL FEEDINGS

In late-stage CF, around 4,000 calories can be burned in a day just from the effort of breathing. Unless you are a big fan of the fast-food chains, it's nearly impossible to consume that many calories in a single day, every day. Trying to meet the daily caloric needs often required can be more than just a challenge. The need for supplemental nutrition and calories that cannot be obtained through food might become a necessity. There are several ways of adding these extra daily calories. Supplemental shakes, such as Ensure or Skandishakes, pack a lot of calories into a small can. But drinking the shakes every day still requires an effort. Popular today as a way to gain this extra boost in nutrition is the gastrostomy tube, or g-tube, which is inserted in the belly. David Hardy, Veronica Villarreal, and Maggie Sheehan all had their g-tubes placed as adolescents and have been very happy with the results.

"I was in the hospital at the time the decision was made to give me a g-tube and I was very sick. I was 11½ years old and I weighed only sixty-one pounds! I had stopped eating because I was very, very tired and didn't have an appetite. My doctors, my parents, and I had a meeting to discuss the issue of getting a g-tube since I had a history of poor weight gain. I did not want to get it, but my opinion (and tears) didn't count for much. My doctors and my parents made the decision. We negotiated and the doctors said that if I grew enough and could keep enough weight on, then when I turn 16, I can get the g-tube removed. I'm only 15 now, but I have already grown to be taller than my mom. I am five feet seven and my weight has been as high as

73

130 (upon my last hospital release). It flexes a bit. I am probably between 120 and 125 right now.

"I completely take care of my g-tube and the preparation of my nighttime feedings myself. I also check the g-tube to make sure the water is in the balloon, and I change the g-tube whenever it needs to be done, although it broke once when I was in class in the eighth grade. It was so gross (and smelly) to have my lunch leaking out of my stomach onto my shirt. Talk about embarrassing! It was one of my worst experiences!

"Being able to grow and gain weight are the only benefit of having a g-tube. And not having my mom and doctors on my back even more than they are now about eating more." On the down side, David has a long list of honest grievances against his g-tube. "The disfigurement to my body is the worst thing. I don't like that I have to swim with a t-shirt on and that I'm uncomfortable changing my shirt in P.E. at school. I don't like feeling like I have to be secretive. I worry about people seeing the bump on my stomach and having to answer their questions. I don't like being tethered to the IV pole at night. I worry about the balloon breaking and coming out when I'm in public. I don't like getting the feeding and tubing ready at night because that lengthens my bedtime preparation by about twenty minutes. (I hate to bother my mom to do it for me.) I don't sleep as well because of the tubing getting tangled in my body. I don't even hear the alarm telling me it is kinked or finished, so my mom has to come across the hall and turn it off in the middle of each night. I don't like that I have to deal with traveling with the feeding equipment or not doing the feeding when I'm away from home."—David Hardy, 15, Modesto, California

With humor, David asks, "Shall I go on?" Yet, when asked what he would tell other teens in regard to getting a g-tube, David firmly states, "It sucks, but do it anyway!"

ANOTHER BOOK WORTH READING

The Spirit of Lo: An Ordinary Family's Extraordinary Journey by Terry Detrich and Don Detrich (Tulsa: Mind Matters, 2000) is a touching story of a loving family's struggle to raise a child who has cystic fibrosis.

"I had my g-tube placed when I was 14 years old and weighed only seventy-two pounds. I had struggled with my weight for years. I was drinking extra calories, sometimes up to three shakes a day. After a while, I just got sick of eating and drinking so much. My doctors suggested the NG-tube (nasogastric tube) when I was 12. I tried it twice and both times I hated it. So I went back to drinking my shakes. Two years after trying the NG-tube, I just could not eat anymore. During a hospital stay, my medical team suggested the g-tube. They gave me all the information I needed about it and I was all for it. At that time, there was nobody I could talk to or ask questions of. All the patients who had g-tubes on my hospital floor were babies. So based on the information my doctor gave me, I decided to get it. I made the decision all on my own and told my parents I was getting a g-tube. They knew I needed it, and they completely supported my decision. It's probably one of the biggest decisions I've made in my life, so far.

"I don't have much of a routine in terms of caring for my g-tube. I just make sure to check it every morning and turn it a couple times during the day, like a pierced earring. And after I do my feeding, I flush it with warm water. And about twice a year, I replace my g-tube with a new one.

"I think there are a few benefits. I don't have to worry about putting it in at night and taking it out every morning like the NG-tube. And gaining weight is the best benefit. I no longer have to eat so much.

"The thing that I dislike about having the g-tube is that I can't lie on my stomach for long periods of time. After a while it starts to really bother me.

"I would tell teens first to consider all their options. And if they still want the g-tube, then I highly recommend it."—Veronica Villarreal, 24, Northbrook, Illinois

Maggie Sheehan got her g-tube when she was 9 years old. The decision was made by her parents, her doctors, and Maggie herself because of Maggie's failure to gain weight. Maggie was tired of her parents' constant badgering to eat. And in truth, even at 9 years old, Maggie was getting sicker. At 16, Maggie calls it her "lifesaver" because the g-tube "takes the pressure off of eating when she doesn't feel like it," says her mom, Kerry. By doing an extra can of nutritional supplement here and there Maggie can add calories if she's been sick.

The only thing Maggie truly dislikes about her g-tube, now that she is a teenager, is that she doesn't like it when she is wearing a bathing suit. "However," explains her mom, "she only wears bikinis." It really isn't a big deal otherwise, her mother says, proudly stating that Maggie never complains about having it.

"If a teenager needs it, I would encourage him or her to get one," says Maggie. "It becomes routine like everything else with CF."

GET MOVING

In addition to the bland diet children were once forced to eat, doctors used to strongly advise children with CF to take it easy. Few kids were allowed to play sports or participate in gym classes at school. It was believed that the children who had CF were too weak or frail to exert themselves and that they should preserve their energy.

Did You Know?
Rosie O'Donnell's young nephew, Joey, has CF. Rosie supports the Great Strides Walk-a-Thon, a fundraiser for the Cystic Fibrosis Foundation.[10]

Today's doctors have a better handle on all of this. They agree that exercise in conjunction with a nutritional diet improves lung strength and increases resistance to lung infection, thereby improving lung function. In addition to traditional exercise and sports, playing a musical instrument (one that is blown into, of course) can also help improve lung strength. All of this, along with the improvements in medications and airway clearance techniques, has done a great deal to improve the lives of those who have cystic fibrosis.

CHALLENGING THE TEEN YEARS

The teen years can be difficult under any circumstances, but add cystic fibrosis to the mix and you are dealing with some

"I love to work out, swim, and bowl, if my strength permits it." —Jessica Hawk-Manus

"I try to exercise every day. I'm working up to a thirty-minute aerobic workout every day and a twelve-minute strength-training/muscle-toning workout three times a week. I'm also expected to mow the lawn." —James Lawlor, 17

"I love marching. I have been doing it since senior year in high school. I don't actually play an instrument. I am in the color guard. I remember telling my mother that I have never felt as healthy as I did during the semesters in which I marched. When I entered college, I tried out and I made it, but had to quit because I was sick. I ended up struggling the whole semester with lung infection and finally did IVs that winter. It was a tough decision for me to have worked so hard and then give up, but it was the right decision. Had I pushed myself, I might not have made it through the semester, and school is very important to me. I had a knee injury the next fall, but finally made it back my junior year and have been happy ever since. I got sick toward the end of my junior year and had to miss a few games, but my instructor was supportive and I had other ways to take part in the performances. This fall (2003) will be my third and final semester marching, as I will be leaving Western for my internship in December. I will definitely miss marching. Not only is it a wonderful way for me to exercise (we have two-hour rehearsals five to six days a week), but it is also a release for me. It is a way for me to forget all about my day, to hang out with so many exciting people, and to hear wonderful music. Music is the universal language. No matter who you are or what you do, music can open your heart and free your mind." —Jackie Goryl, 23

"I used to do gymnastics until I was 13, and alternate between squash, jogging, and gym in high school. For the last one and a half years, however, I feel as if my physical abilities have declined. This is due to the fact that my chest feels closed up and tight more frequently, and I can't get my peak flow to what it used to be. I still try to make a point of going to the gym three times a week and do weight-bearing exercises and as much cardio as I can cope with." —Alice Vosloo, 19

"I've been cheerleading since sixth grade. I'll be trying out again next October for basketball season. We practice two days a week from November through February. The basketball games are on the weekends. The expectations on me are the same as for the other girls. I also used to dance when I was little and in eighth grade I was in show choir, which is a dancing and singing performance group." —Maggie Sheehan, 15

"When I was really little I was very active in sports. In high school I stopped growing, and I was really short; I was about five feet one. So I stopped competing. Now I'm five feet six. I live in Colorado, which is great for physical activity. I love to go mountain hiking, rock climbing, and snowboarding. I recently climbed to the peak of a 14,000-foot mountain. We started at the 11,000-foot mark and climbed up another five miles. That was a huge accomplishment for me! I'm really excited about having done that!" —Chad Lucci, 25, who believes his healthy attitude accounts for his healthy lifestyle serious challenges. While it is unknown for certain exactly why, some people who have cystic fibrosis see a decline in their health during their teen years. Puberty makes many demands on the body as it changes a child into an adult. These demands can be stressful. Some teens make it through just fine, obviously, and live on into their 20s, 30s, or even longer. Others make it through, but their lungs sustain too much damage and they die in their 20s. (There are also still those who don't make it through—or even to—their teen years at all.) Knowing this adds even more stress to the already stressed preteen or teenager. After all, besides having CF, you are wondering if you'll get an A in algebra class, wondering if your hair and clothes are right, wondering whether you will have a date for the prom, and wondering where you might consider going to college. All of the things that worry the typical teenager are also worrisome to the teen who has cystic fibrosis. Having CF just adds to the worries.

In addition to the daily challenges to meet all of your body's physical and nutritional needs, there are also mental and emotional challenges to living with cystic fibrosis. Jessica, James, Alice, Janelle, Jackie, and Chad share their biggest challenges as teens and young adults with CF.

"For me it was keeping the whole CF thing a secret. I didn't want anyone to know I was different, although folks found out after I bled out internally the first time from my liver. Also, I had trouble with my bowels. I would have to go to the bathroom at least once every hour and the teachers would give me a hard time about it. At the time, I also had severe gas, which was terrifying to me. After my liver transplant though, my bowels are normal and my gas is normal as well."—Jessica Hawk-Manus

"I guess my biggest challenge would have to be fitting CF and everything that goes along with it in with a 'normal life,' although I'm glad that things are going as well as they are."
—James Lawlor

"Trying to be normal and fitting in with my friends."—Alice Vosloo

"During my teens, I would have to say it was trying to get through school when I was never there. It is really hard to do if your teachers are not willing to make accommodations. I lucked out; most of my teachers were great. Also during my teens I lost quite a few friends with CF, which forced me to consider my own mortality. It forced me to deal with a lot of different feelings. I went through a bout of depression, which I think is normal when you lose people. I had to come to terms with that and my CF. I had to accept the fact that CF does kill people, which I hadn't really believed until I saw it. Ultimately I had to come to terms with the fact that CF probably will kill me, which I had never really believed. In college a friend of mine with CF and I lived together. We both went through a morbid phase of planning our own funerals. I was surprised when we talked about it after we had lost a couple of mutual friends. I also had to deal with a bit of survivor guilt. I felt bad that I was healthier than people who were younger than me. I still deal with survivor guilt a little but not like I used to."
—Janelle Benitez, 25, Michigan

"For me, fitting in was very hard. I was always small, and I was embarrassed of my CF. I was always wondering what people thought about me and tried everything I could to be normal. Teenage years are hard on everyone and adding CF or anything else that makes you different can make these years unbearable."
—Jackie Goryl, 23

"I don't think any teenager can say they've not done regrettable things. So I was a normal teenager in that aspect. But there were two sides of me. There was the responsible side that knew I had to be mature and take care of myself, and there was the cynical, rebellious side that would wreak havoc on my own life and on my family, as teens are known to do. It was hard to be a teenager knowing I would most likely live to be 30 at most. I wasn't dealing with this very well. I went through a self-destructive phase because I figured I was going to die anyway.

At 15 or 16 all I could see was that I didn't have much of a future, so it didn't matter what I did. I couldn't have said this all so plainly at the time and would in fact have denied these reasons for my bad behavior. This was all very hard on my mom. I'm sure I damaged my health with all the things I did as a teenager. I know I probably shortened my life a little. But my philosophy is to enjoy life. I'm not really a long-term thinker, and I especially wasn't back then. I've always just tried to get the most out of my life, both as a teenager and now."—Chad Lucci, 25

Getting through ages 13 through 19 can be rough at times, even under the best of circumstances. Add the challenges of cystic fibrosis and these years can be downright difficult. Some teens who have CF are able to take it all in stride. They are so used to dealing with their CF that it is simply not an issue. For others, the issue is great. How a teenager deals with his or her own illness is as individual as the person. Many teens and young adults hate coughing and spitting out mucus in front of other people, and they go to great lengths not to do it. They are worried that other people will be "grossed out." For some, it might seem easier not to be around friends at all. Or they spend limited time with friends and then try to wait until they are alone to do all of their coughing. This is hardly a healthy situation, yet coughing in front of friends is a common concern for young people who have CF. But the truth of the matter is, the coughing is what helps keep your lungs clean. If you don't cough, bacteria and germs are making themselves comfy and cozy in the warm, moist mucus in your lungs. They grab a bite to eat while they're in there, too, destroying your healthy lung tissue. Yuck! Cough it *out*! (Don't swallow it, either. You don't want that mess filling up your belly.) Keep a supply of tissues handy or excuse

Did You Know?
NASCAR racer Kimberly Myers had CF. You can read about her achievements at personal.nbnet .nb.ca/normap/CF.htm.

yourself to the bathroom. Just get that junk out of your lungs. It's a matter of life and death.

Another common complaint made by many young people who have CF has to do with eating. Often teens who have CF, especially teenage girls, complain that their parents and doctors are always trying to make them eat. One young lady says that her mother packs her "all this food for lunch and when I don't eat it, she goes nuts. I'm sick of it. I just don't want to eat. Nothing tastes good, and I'm just not hungry anyway. You can make me do a lot of things, but you can't make me eat if I don't want to." Both the teen who has CF and the parent trying to force the food issue become very frustrated as they continue to butt heads over the situation. Eventually it becomes an issue of control. Everyone loses when the battle with CF is lost.

As you have already read, proper nutrition is a key element in warding off lung infections. While there is no easy answer to the issue of eating, there are some things that should be addressed. First, despite what you might say, it's unlikely that you actually are not hungry. It is more likely that you are trying to gain some control over your own life in the only way you know how. Your parents can insist that you do your therapy, go to the doctor, and take your medicines, but, no, they can't force you to eat. The hardest thing for a parent to do is watch his or her child hurt him- or herself. If only your parents could just back off a bit! This is a very sensitive issue and while most often the problem will resolve itself, it can still be very frustrating while it's going on. Indulge your parents; try eating a little. It won't kill you. On the other hand, *not* eating can cause serious damage to your organs, including your brain, and it can lower your resistance to infection. If it's control you are looking for, this is the best opportunity to take control in a positive way. Help yourself to be the healthiest you possible.

Yet another issue for many teens and young adults who have CF is embarrassment over letting anyone besides immediate family and best friends witness a therapy session. They don't think people will understand what they are doing, and they are again afraid to "gross them out." For some this is just a simple need for privacy. But for others the worry is more far-reaching. One young man said, "I am afraid to go to college. What if I do not have privacy to do my nebs and Vest? What will my friends think of me?"

While the need for privacy might seem overwhelming for some teens, perhaps the need to treat their CF should be moved to the forefront. Your body needs medications and therapies. There is nothing to be ashamed of here. It might seem rather frightening to open yourself up and share the details of cystic fibrosis with your friends. But the outcome could surprise you. Explain to your friends what you are doing, and tell them why you have to do it. Encourage them to ask you questions. You might eventually wish to invite them to join you in a game of cards or a video game to help pass the time while you do your treatments. If you are considering going away to college, consider requesting a single dorm room. While most universities don't offer single dorm rooms to freshmen, under these circumstances, most universities will make exceptions.

A universal theme among all teens is fitting in. "I just want to be like everyone else." For those who have CF, this simple statement can take on a deeper meaning than just wanting to look like and dress like your friends. You don't want to have to stop and cough. You don't want to have to sit down and rest a moment in the middle of gym class. You don't want to have to be home by a certain time so that you can do your treatment before you go to bed. You just want to hang out and not think about being sick. The fact of the matter is that you have cystic fibrosis. Hiding this fact will do you no good. Sure, it might cramp your style to think about what your body needs all the time, but taking care of yourself is what will actually allow you to "be like everyone else" and have fun for another day. Ignoring CF so that you will fit in and not be seen as different can cause serious problems with your health. Unfortunately, it is not uncommon for a teenager to seem by all appearances to be as healthy as his or her friends, but because he or she doesn't take proper measures to treat the symptoms of cystic fibrosis, he or she drastically shortens what could have been a much longer life.

This is exactly what happened to Talia*. She always seemed so healthy. She looked healthy. People who didn't know her would never have guessed she was sick. She partied with her

high school friends, stayed
out late, and drank
alcoholic beverages with
her classmates— all
typical teenager
stuff. While these
behaviors can cause
problems for a healthy
teenager, they can be
deadly for a teen who has
CF. This is especially true
when these behaviors are

Did You Know?
Country singer and songwriter
Tammy Cochran dedicated her song
"Angels in Waiting" to her two
brothers, Shawn and Alan, who died
of CF at ages 14 and 23.[11]

prioritized over getting enough sleep, eating properly, taking
your meds, and doing your daily therapy. Pair that with a
strong dose of denial, as in, "See, I can do everything my friends
do. I'm not sick!" and you could be seriously jeopardizing your
own health. Your lifestyle, your denial of CF, and your strong
desire to be like everyone else might backfire once and for all, as
it did for Talia. Seemingly healthy, energetic, and strong as a
horse, Talia surprised everyone: she died when she was just 17
years old.

CHALLENGING THE YOUNG ADULT YEARS

Some of those who shared their experiences about the
challenges of being a teen with CF are now young adults. For
Alice, Jackie, Jessica, and Janelle, the challenges have changed
to some extent.

"The greatest challenges for me now are taking responsibility
of my health, especially regarding the choices I make
concerning my future; hoping to find a husband one day who
will support and encourage me; and eventually learning to cope
with a full-time job after I've finished studying, and still have
energy left for exercising, and so forth."—Alice Vosloo

"Relationships are always hard for me, especially now that I
am getting older and having longer and more serious
relationships. While I have not had a boyfriend scared off by

the CF or refuse to see me again because of it, they just don't understand and can't relate to me. CF affects every aspect of life, and now that I am becoming more independent, I am seeing firsthand just how much it influences my decisions. I can't go out and have fun every night like most of the people my age; otherwise, I pay for it the next day (antibiotics and alcohol don't mix, nor do smoke-filled clubs and CF lungs). I have responsibilities that most 21-year-olds don't have. I have lots of doctor appointments and am probably the most informed 21-year-old when it comes to health insurance. Sometimes I wish I could be one of those college kids without a care in the world."—Jackie Goryl, 23

"Keeping up with everyone else is hard. Not being able to work has been incredibly hard for me. Every time I try to work I end up being out sick more than I am at the actual job."—Jessica Hawk-Manus

"As a young adult I still deal with some survivor guilt. I also had to come to terms with the fact that I am not going to have children. I know I could physically have children, but I am choosing not to. I don't feel I could provide a stable environment for a child if I am sick all the time. Also, I don't feel it is fair to the child. He wouldn't have a normal upbringing, and there is a good chance I might not be around to see him grow up. I would also be afraid of having a child with CF. I would feel terribly bad if that happened. Plus, children are physically demanding for healthy people. It took me a long process to get to the decision, but I believe it is the right one for me. My other big challenge is a fairly normal one. I can't decide what I want to be when I grow up! I have way too many interests."—Janelle Benitez, Michigan

Did You Know?
"The Cystic Fibrosis Foundation supports and accredits more than 115 CF care centers nationwide that provide high-quality, specialized care for those with CF."[12]

NOTES

1. Frank Deford, *Alex: The Life of a Child* (Nashville: Rutledge Hill Press, 1997), 37.

2. Patricia Beck Hoff, Donald Eitzman, and Josef Neu, *Neonatal and Pediatric Respiratory Care* (St. Louis: Mosby-Year Book, 1993).

3. Canadian Cystic Fibrosis Foundation, www.cysticfibrosis .ca/page.asp?id=82; Earthlink, search.earthlink.net/search?q=dornase; and Medicine.net, www.medicinenet.com/dornase_alpha/article.htm.

4. Cystic Fibrosis Foundation, cff.org/about_cf/what_is_cf.cfm?CFID=1619012&CFTOKEN=8499 1526.

5. NIDDK: Cystic fibrosis research directions, www.niddk .nih.gov.health/endo/pubs/cystic/cystic.htm.

6. NIDDK: Cystic fibrosis research directions.

7. American Biosystems, classes.kumc.edu/cahe/respcared/ cybercas/cysticfibrosis/tracpurp.html.

8. American Biosystems.

9. Norma Kennedy Plourde's Cystic Fibrosis website, www3.nbnct.nb.ca/normap/cfhistory.htm.

10. Norma Kennedy Plourde's Cystic Fibrosis website.

11. Cystic Fibrosis Foundation.

12. Cystic Fibrosis Foundation.

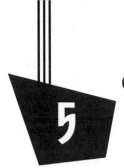

Good Days and Bad Days

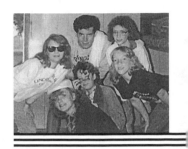

It rained a lot at camp. We had wet feet almost all week that first year. But we had fun despite the rain. Everyone was the same at camp. The "outsiders" would have been the ones who did not have cystic fibrosis, rather than the ones who did. But there were no outsiders. Just a bunch of kids enjoying the summer, rain and all, and hoping for just enough sunshine to warm our faces and allow for time out on a rowboat, a jump on the trampoline, a pick-up game of basketball or volleyball after dinner, or maybe just a few quiet moments lying atop a picnic table under the summer sky. At CF camp, there were mostly good days, because everyone was the same.

"**I** have good days and bad days." That was the way Kimberlee Pilarczyk described her life with cystic fibrosis. Kimberlee lived just long enough to celebrate her 21st birthday. Her life was full and fun, and she lived it to the limits. At 20, Kimberlee was attending college, majoring in sociology and minoring in criminology. She planned to work in the jail system. She was holding down a job, dating, and enjoying an active social life. She was a fine example of living life to its fullest despite a life-threatening illness. Her attitude was 100 percent in favor of putting it all out there.

While not a contagious disease, cystic fibrosis is still a disease. The word alone conjures up all sorts of images of sick people and hospitals and medicines. But the fact that CF is a chronic illness, one that must be managed and lived with,

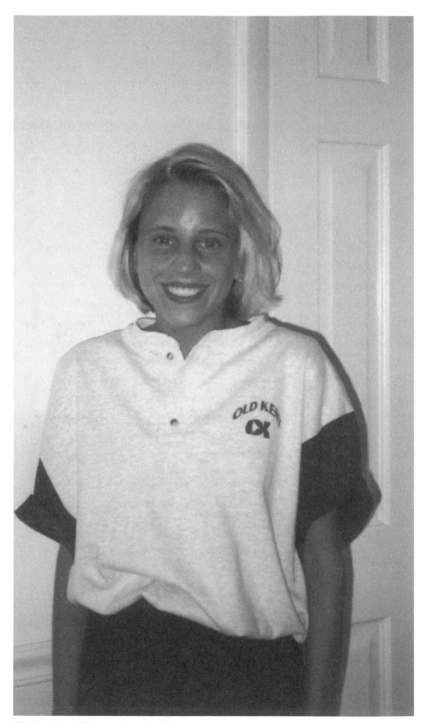

Kimberlee Pilarczyk, age 20

presents certain challenges on the social scene as well. There is a wide spectrum of how people who have cystic fibrosis deal with their illness in social situations.

Everyone who knows 18-year-old Katie Kocelko knows she has CF. After two double lung transplants and countless days, weeks, and even months of school missed, how could Katie keep her illness a secret? By contrast, Trina* never told anyone she had CF. In the final hours of her life, her family decided Trina would rather succumb to cystic fibrosis than be on oxygen in front of people she knew. Whatever anyone decides regarding the disclosure of his or her illness is, of course, his or her own decision. However, evidence shows that dealing with the disease outright generally leads to better overall health. After all, it is much easier to take your medicines and cough in front of your friends than it is to go to great lengths to hide all the necessities of maintaining your health.

> **Oh this monster**
> **Creeping inside me**
> **It growls in hunger**
> **Ravaging my body**
>
> **The embarrassment**
> **It causes me**
> **Making me cry**
>
> **Will there ever be an end**
> **Or maybe some hope**
> **I need a friend**
> **To help me cope**
>
> **No one else knows**
> **That's why I'm alone**
> **Letting me be**
> **In this world of my own**
> **—Leah K., teen with CF**

Kimberlee Pilarczyk was straightforward about her disease. When talking about her current boyfriend, she said, "He understands pretty much. I tell him. . . . That's probably the hardest thing, I think, to tell people that you have CF. They don't understand. Most people don't know what it is. They don't want to ask questions because they don't want to feel like they are bothering you. I usually start out telling people I have asthma (which I do have). Then when I get to know them, I tell them I have CF because by then it's obvious that asthma wouldn't be as bad as what I have."

Kimberlee said that she'd rather have people ask her "a million questions" about having CF than leave wondering what it is, not understanding it, and not wanting to talk to her about it. "I try to explain it," Kimberlee said, "I tell people to imagine when they have a cold and it goes to their chest. They say 'Oh' and I say, 'well, I feel like that all the time.' I tell them I have good days and I have bad days."

"A good day is when I wake up without a headache," Kimberlee said, "and I can walk through my house without breathing heavy. Or I can go out and have a good time. A bad day for me is when I wake up with a headache. I usually know right then that I'm going to have a lousy day, and that every time that I even exert myself with the least amount of energy I am going to be out of breath. The headache is probably from a lack of oxygen. I usually have five bad days and two good days in a given week."

It would seem that on a good day, all would have been fine, and on a bad day, Kimberlee might have had to stay home and rest. But Kimberlee said, no, on a bad day, "I just get dressed and I go [to work]. If I were to call in sick for every bad day, there are a lot of days that I wouldn't be doing anything. I've called in sick one time," she says, amazingly, "and that was because when I woke up I felt like everything was spinning, and I was pale and gray. I felt lousy. I couldn't walk or do anything. I called the doctor and he said to go to the hospital. My mom took me right away. My oxygen level was 74 percent when normal is in the high nineties. I don't know what mine is normally, but that day it was so low I had to stay in the hospital."

Kimberlee said that people at her office knew she had CF because she felt it was necessary to explain so that they would understand why she went into the hospital. She appreciated that her coworkers understood when she didn't feel well and gave her time to sit down and catch her breath now and then.

For many, one of the toughest things to deal with when you have a disease like cystic fibrosis is sharing this information. For some, this part is easy. If you look sick, if you cough a lot, if you frequently miss school or work, an explanation is almost required. But for others, especially those who look remarkably healthy despite their illness, it seems simpler to keep it to themselves. Often whether or not a person who has CF shares information about his or her disease is determined by his or her parents. Statements made by parents such as, "We want her to have a normal life, so we don't tell people she has CF," although certainly well meaning, could in fact backfire horribly.

While the idea of living as normal a life as possible is a good one, doing so by pretending not to have CF will not amount to anything positive. Too many young people who have CF get caught up in appearances. They don't want to cough in front of their friends, or they don't want to be seen taking their pills. And they most certainly wouldn't ever wish to be caught doing their respiratory therapy. But all of this hiding often leads to self-neglect. If you can't take proper care of yourself at all times, your health will suffer. Inevitably, it is the ones who work the hardest to hide their disease who suffer the most and die the most quickly and unexpectedly. By not acknowledging and taking control of the disease, they actually allow it to take control of them.

BUT, SEE, I'M NOT THAT SICK—A LESSON IN DENIAL

Martin* was so afraid to do his therapy because, he said, he and his sister Becki* never did much therapy when they were little. But when Becki got older and CF started to catch up with her, she did everything the doctors told her to do. She did her nebulizers and her chest therapy twice or more every day. But she died when she was only 18 years old anyway. Martin was afraid that if he started doing his treatments every day, it would mean that he was as sick as Becki had been. He thought for sure this would mean he would die, too. He desperately wanted to prove that he was much healthier than his older sister had been. Unfortunately for Martin and for others who think this way, the opposite was true. Relatively healthy as far as CF goes, Martin didn't do his treatments and he died before he reached his 26th birthday. Had Martin taken control of his CF instead of letting his fear of CF control him, perhaps he would still be alive today.

WHAT TO TELL YOUR FRIENDS . . . OR NOT

"When I was little I used to just tell people I had asthma. Then later on if I learned I could trust them, I told them I had CF. The asthma part was true, actually. The kids didn't get mad at me because I lied because, really, I just hadn't told them everything. When I was in fourth grade one of my classmates was a real tattletale. I made the mistake of telling her I had CF and the next thing I knew, everyone in fourth grade knew. It was okay. Everyone pretty much knew already. My teachers knew every year, and they usually told the kids if I didn't. Usually, the first time I went into the hospital they'd ask [the teacher] why I was gone so long. Then when I'd come back to school, the kids would tell me what they knew about my absence. I had one best friend back then who I could really trust. I told her everything. She knew when I was really sick, and she knew all about the medical procedures I had to undergo. Actually, she thought it was pretty cool to have a friend with CF.

"Now I'm about to go away to college, and I'm prepared to answer questions when I get there. In high school I didn't want to tell the whole world that I had cystic fibrosis and that I'd had a [double lung] transplant because I thought maybe I'd be treated differently or looked at differently by the kids. It's nothing to be embarrassed about, though, so I'd rather just tell people. When I notice people watching me take my pills or something I tell them [why]."—Katie Kocelko, 18

But telling a friend, especially a boyfriend or a girlfriend, can be a frightening task.

"Most of my old friends from school knew that I have CF. I grew up with them, and their parents told them about my CF when they were small. We never talked about it though. I'm still looking for the right moment to tell my new university friends, but I keep putting it off because I don't really know how to tell them. I can't exactly go, 'Hey, by the way, I've got a life-threatening disease called cystic fibrosis, any questions?'"
—Alice Vosloo, South Africa

◉

"One of my friends cried," says Leah K. about her experiences telling her friends she has cystic fibrosis. "One of my friends couldn't have cared less and changed the subject, and one has been so interested that she wants to work with people who have CF."—Leah K., 22, Orion, Michigan

◉

"Most of my close friends know about my CF. My best friend has known since we were in junior high school, and she has been extremely supportive of me. Whenever I was in the hospital or needed surgery, she was right there for me. She has been there every step of the way. I tell most people out of necessity. I am more open about my CF than I used to be, but I still don't go around telling everyone; I don't want people to treat me differently. Usually when I need IVs or I am pretty sick, I will tell a friend if he or she asks why I am so sick.

"Most of my boyfriends have known. Most were understanding and supportive. There have been times when I have ended a relationship because the guy just didn't seem to understand about CF. I don't want a hero who feels the need to save me every time I am sick, but I do need someone who doesn't feel bothered or forced to visit me in the hospital or wait with me while I do a nebulizer treatment. He should do that because he wants to and because he supports me. One particular boyfriend would play Nintendo 64 games with me while I did my treatments. It became a ritual for us. Relationships are hard because I am getting to a time in my life where I am beginning to look for 'The One.' At the same time, it is hard for me to knowingly put someone through any pain. CF will not get easier, and it will take its toll on me as well as my future husband. Sometimes I feel it is unfair to put that person through that pain, whoever he may be."—Jackie Goryl

93

Janelle Benitez* looks back on her high school years and reports:

"In high school I kept my CF a secret, which, in retrospect, I think was a bad idea. I couldn't really connect with people because I always felt like I was hiding something. Now I am very open about it. I don't really care who knows. In general I prefer people to know. It's not the first thing I tell people, however. Generally, I wait until someone asks about my coughing. Then I just say I have a lung disease called cystic fibrosis. I tell them that it's genetic and that they can't get it from me. I explain that basically I get lung infections like pneumonia, and then I have to go to the hospital for IV antibiotics, and that other than that it just makes me cough a lot.

"I am pretty open about it, so people usually feel comfortable asking questions, which I tell them to do. My close friends know more about it, and I found out later on that they went and did research on it. I think it's pretty cool that they were concerned and cared enough to want to learn more. Not a lot of people do that. Most people who don't really know me just say, 'Okay.' They usually don't bring it up again unless I am sick. Then when I have to go to the hospital they ask again. I find most people just want to make sure they can't get anything from me. Once they understand that, they really don't think about it or care much about it. Really, why should they? After all, it doesn't affect them. The people who ask questions are generally the ones who want to get to know me better.

"My boyfriend knows I have CF. I don't know how someone could hide it from a boyfriend or girlfriend, but I guess you could. Everyone I have dated for more than one or two dates has known at the very least that I have health problems. In high school my boyfriend knew. I actually called him for the first time from the hospital! He was curious what all the noises in the background were, so I just told him. He drove an hour the next day to visit me. I have found if people are worth knowing, it doesn't change things when they find out I have CF. My current boyfriend is wonderful. We live together and he is great with therapy. He sits with me and keeps me company while I do it. He is a light sleeper, but he claims to sleep through my coughing at night unless it is really bad. If it's bad enough that I wake up from it, I will usually find him standing next to me holding a glass of water. He also doesn't get grossed out by my mucus. What more could I ask for?! He has driven me three hours to the hospital because I was too sick to drive myself and stayed overnight in a chair to be with me. He never gets upset when I am really hungry at a restaurant, but I'm only able to eat a few bites because my chest is too tight to eat. Basically, he's almost perfect, but don't tell him that!"

"My friends and classmates all know I have CF. My mom came and talked to the class when I was younger to explain about CF."—Krystal Freake, 16

Simple as that.

ANOTHER BOOK WORTH READING

In *Breathing for a Living: A Memoir* (New York: Hyperion, 2003), Laura Rothenberg writes about her wait for a double lung transplant and her fight against rejection following the transplant, all while trying to earn a college degree. Written honestly and straightforwardly, 21-year-old Laura's life is as much like any other typical college student's as it can be, except where cystic fibrosis counts.

From an early age, Kerry Sheehan says, her daughter Maggie, now almost 16, never made a big deal about her CF. When Maggie was 7, Kerry said:

"Maggie had a sleepover last night with her little friend Melissa. I'm sure Melissa knows that Maggie was in the hospital and stuff but she said, 'What are you doing to her?' I was doing her pounding. I said, 'Maggie, tell her,' but Maggie was really tired so I just said, 'She's got junky lungs, and we're going to get that junk out and have her spit it out.' And we just did it. It was just nothing, not made into a big deal or anything."

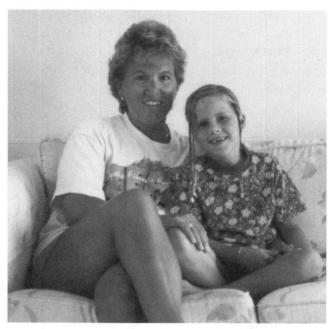

Maggie Sheehan at age 7 with her mom, Kerry

When Maggie was 7 years old she was already quite matter-of-fact about her disease and treated it as a nuisance more than anything else:

"A lot of my friends, like the people next door and a lot of people on my block, and a lot of my friends that I know at school, know I have CF. Sometimes they want to know stuff and I'm like, 'Oh please, will you stop!' When I'm trying to take my pills at school and the kids ask me questions, I'm like, 'Do I have to tell you?' They ask things like, 'Can we get it?' or, 'What do your pills taste like?' or, 'Why do you have to go in the hospital?' All different kinds of questions. They can't get CF because you can only get it when you're born. You can only get certain stuff that you're born with, but sometimes, like a cold, you can just get from other people. I tell them that. I don't really think they know what it's called, but I'm pretty sure they do. [When I was in the hospital] one friend sent me all these cards, and I think she knew what I was in for because she wrote all these questions."—Maggie Sheehan

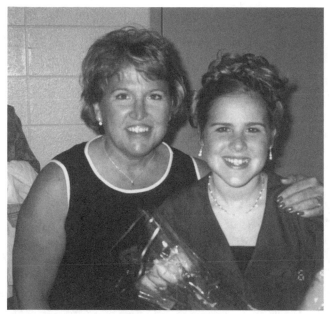

Maggie Sheehan in 2002, at age 14, with her mom

CF: AN ASSET?

Sometimes the fact that someone knows about your CF can be your best asset of all.

> "I have CF to thank for my husband. I'd had quite a fair share of boyfriends but was dumped most of the time because they couldn't handle my health problems. I met my husband Casey at the hospital. I was still in high school when I found out about my liver problem. Casey worked alongside my liver transplant doctor in the GI lab. I didn't get to really know Casey, just talked to him while they were prepping me for an endoscopy, which I'd had a million of! Years later I moved to Nashville, and Casey had been keeping up with me through my doctor. Of course, I didn't know that. One evening after I got home from work the phone rang and it was Casey. He wanted to go to lunch some time. The rest is history!"—Jessica Hawk-Manus

What and how and even *if* you decide to tell your friends, coworkers, or potential dates comes down to personal choice. However, being as straightforward as you can about your disease is your best option.

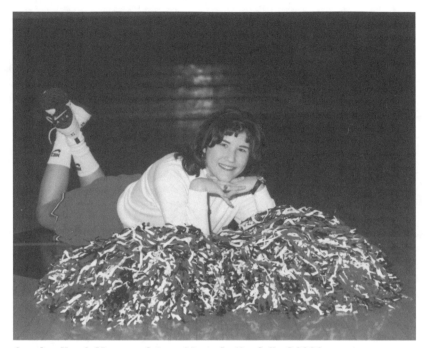

Jessica Hawk-Manus, pictured here in the fall of 1996, was a cheerleader in high school.

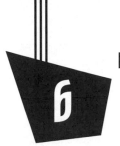

Living and Laughing

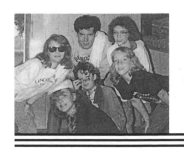

By the final evening of my first week at CF camp I knew I had met some amazing children and young people. In seven days, my life had been touched and changed in many ways. I knew I would be returning to camp the following summer because my experience was too good and too important to be a one-shot deal. My new friends and I sat around in the Fun Lodge (it was raining again so we had to forgo the traditional campfire), and one of the older campers told a story about warm fuzzies. Then we passed around our own warm fuzzies, short pieces of colored yarn that we tied to a long piece of yarn that was hanging like a necklace around each of our necks. With each warm fuzzy we knotted, we said something nice to the person whose necklace we were helping create. It was usually simple things like, "It was so great to meet you this year," or "Thank you for doing my therapy every morning," or "You really made me laugh on skit night." One of the questions I was asked over and over that evening was, "Are you coming back next year?" I had not thought about the answer prior to the first time I answered, "Absolutely!" There was no way I was going to miss out on this experience. But I never asked the question back to any of the campers that night because the answer in some cases was so painfully obvious. No, some of the kids would not be returning the following summer because they would not live that long.

I loved CF camp and I loved being able to visit my camp friends when they checked into the hospital, which was about four blocks from my house. I was always trying to push buttons or turn off beeping IVs; I asked quite a few questions of the respiratory therapists who came in to give my friends their breathing treatments. I always said hello to the doctors in hopes that they would eventually recognize me from one patient room to the next. But try as I might, I eventually came to realize that visiting was not enough for me. I wanted to help take care of the kids who had CF on a regular basis, not just as a visitor who brought pizza, ice cream, and videos, and not just one week a year at camp. I wanted to work at the hospital. I returned to school and earned a degree in respiratory care so that I could work at the very hospital in which so many of my camp friends were treated.

I think my patients would have been surprised by my excitement over their admissions. No, I was never happy that they were sick. But I was definitely happy to see the kids I knew and cared so much about. It always brightened my workday to know I would get to go in and take care of Katie, Mike, Stephanie, or Veronica. Hospital admissions were routine for my friends. I don't know whether they were upsetting or if they were just taken in stride along with everything else about cystic fibrosis. I do wonder, though, how it might have made any of them feel to know that someone there was excited to see them and so happy to be able to hang out with them and help them get back on their feet.

THE HOSPITAL, AKA CLUB MED FOR CYSTICS

For the general population, thoughts of hospitals are limited. Hospitals are for old people. Hospitals are where women go to have babies. But for those who live with cystic fibrosis, more often than not, the word "hospital" bears great similarity in meaning to the word "home."

Cystic fibrosis is a disease that generally requires a significant amount of maintenance. Regular nebulizer treatments, pills, and therapies do a great deal to maintain the health of those who have CF. But on occasion, and for some more often than for others, this therapy and drug regimen falls short of what the body needs to stay alive. Routine trips to the hospital are required. Known in the CF community as "tune-ups" or "clean outs," these hospital stays typically last from ten to fourteen days. During this time, strong concentrations of IV antibiotics are given in the hopes of killing the bacteria that are causing infection in the lungs. Airway clearance therapy, commonly done at home just twice a day, will be administered by respiratory therapists diligently four or more times a day. Nutrition is monitored and often adjusted. And there are trips to the physical therapy department for muscle strengthening. After all, lying around in bed for two weeks, while relaxing, can sometimes do more damage than good.

For the luckier ones, hospital visits are very infrequent; for most, the average is once or twice a year. But for those whose disease has progressed, hospital stays become more and more regular. They occur maybe every six months for a while, then every four, and then even more often as the time between infections grows shorter and shorter and the need for antibiotics and extra care becomes more and more urgent.

"I'm not hospitalized often; I was in the hospital for CF once this year."
—Krystal Freake, 16

"My first time in the hospital was in 1991. Since then I've been on IV four times but at home, for a number of reasons. The main reason is probably that the public healthcare (provincial hospitals) in South Africa has deteriorated unbelievably. It would be a health risk to go there, and I'd probably come back with new diseases! Unfortunately, private hospitals are very expensive."—Alice Vosloo, 19

"I've been very lucky. I do IV antibiotics about once a year for two weeks, and the past two years I have done them completely on an outpatient basis. Radiology puts in my PICC line, and as long as there aren't any complications, I go home right after. This has been wonderful for me, as I don't have to miss a lot of my classes. The first time I ever had to do IV antibiotics was in sixth grade. I was 12 years old and completely terrified. It was not all that bad, but the fear of the unknown makes everything scary."—Jackie Goryl, 23

(continued)

> "I was first hospitalized with walking pneumonia at the age of 16. Now I am hospitalized an average of seven times a year."—Jessica Hawk-Manus
>
> "I was first hospitalized at 4 weeks old and then not again until I was 4 years old and then not again until I was 11 years old. After that it became a pretty regular thing every three to four months for about a week, followed by a week of home IVs. During my teens and puberty, my hospitalizations became more frequent, and I missed a whole quarter of my senior year of high school. I think the number of days I made it to school was fewer than the days I didn't."—Janelle Benitez
>
> "Luckily I have yet to be hospitalized for CF or anything else (except for a hernia operation as a baby)."—James Lawlor

Because hospital stays become more and more frequent, the relationships between the patients and their caregivers often become intense.

"The healthcare workers throughout my life have been tremendous in trying to help me be my healthiest and my best. I have met a lot of really great people through the unfortunate circumstances of my CF."—Chad Lucci

"I was going through a rough spell healthwise, and I complained to my doctor at one visit that I saw him more regularly than I did some of my friends. His response was, 'I like to think of myself as your friend and not just your doctor.' Since then, he has become a very dear and trusted friend."—Laura Tillman, Northville, Michigan, now almost 57, defied diagnosis until she was 47 years old.

Kerry, mother of 16-year-old Maggie, says that Maggie's hospital stays have always been full of thoughtful gestures on the part of the CF team:

"One doctor used to bring his dog, Barclay, to the hospital on the weekends. He used to take the CF kids (before infection control) to get chocolate shakes across the street from the hospital. Another doctor once got a 'sky box' suite on Easter Sunday and took the CF families to a hockey game. The third doctor on the CF team always brings cinnamon rolls on the weekends she's on call. Once when Maggie was younger, she was in the hospital on Thanksgiving, and one of her respiratory therapists brought her a little plastic box of corn. I think the therapist had asked Maggie what special treat she'd want on the holiday. And then she went out and even decorated the box with Maggie's name."—Kerry Sheehan

Daelynn is the mother of a 9-year-old boy who has cystic fibrosis:

"Billy has not been in the hospital very much, but his CF medical care team is absolutely wonderful. In May, he had to have his first 'tune up' in five years. The whole staff was great. His CF doctor explained everything to Billy before placing his PICC line, and he made sure Billy was ok through the whole procedure. The next morning the nurse from the CF clinic came to visit us in our room. The lady who makes the appointments even brought Billy a present. His medical team has always gone above and beyond what is expected."—Daelynn Williams, New London, Texas

Jeremy Becker still maintains an e-mail correspondence with several of his nurses following his admission to Yale Hospital in March 2003:

"I was admitted for CF and for diabetes, and I was there so long that the nurses were sad for me to go. They said they were going to miss me. That really meant a lot to me."—Jeremy Becker, 25, Beacon Falls, Connecticut

And sometimes the person who does the most and who means the most is not a trained healthcare worker but a family member.

Angela Budnieski had been in the hospital for almost seven weeks in the spring of 2003. She had undergone major surgery and had ballooned from 110 pounds up to 200 pounds due to a combination of medications and complications. She needed help to do everything, even to make the short trip from her hospital bed to the bathroom. She returned home in time to write the following message to her mother in a Mother's Day card:

> Mom,
>
> I just wanted to let you know how important you are to me. I truly appreciate all the time you took off to be with me; I have never felt so loved. I also wanted to tell you I have never felt so close to you as I do now. I love you with all my heart and so much more.
>
> Love, Angie

JENNIFER'S HOME AWAY FROM HOME

Jennifer Cherry was 20 years old when she sat in the teen lounge of Children's Memorial Hospital in Chicago to be interviewed. She was dressed in a typical camp-style outfit of short-shorts and a tie-dyed T-shirt. She talked about her memories of CF camp as well as her very positive experiences as a frequent patient in the hospital.

> "I've been coming into the hospital since I was 12. When I was younger it was fun being here at the same time as a lot of my friends. We used to stay up till three, four, five o'clock in the morning playing cards and watching TV or roaming the halls getting into a lot of trouble! For instance, when new cystics would come in, we'd always initiate them by bringing them down to the morgue! Usually the morgue is locked, but one particular night for some reason the door was unlocked and my friends, Chad and Tina, went in. Tina told a nurse she thought she could trust and the story spread like wildfire! Even though I didn't go in, I was the oldest in the group, so I was the one who got in trouble because I didn't stop them!
>
> "We used to just hang out with each other, sit on each other's beds and watch TV. We were like brothers and sisters. We used to take walks across the street to the gymnasium and play basketball. Then we would get in trouble because we would play so hard that our IVs would come out! We played practical jokes on each other, too. A couple of times my friend

David Bailey got taped to the bed while he was sleeping. It took three rolls of surgical tape! He'd wake up and he couldn't move! We had lots of water fights with big, old 60 cc syringes. John Ozga was the most creative with the syringes. He'd take the tubing from a nebulizer, fill it with water, connect it to the flow meter, and turn the flow meter on. The oxygen from the flow meter would shoot water across the room. We were pretty inventive. My brother Scott's favorite prank was to put Vaseline on the ear of someone's phone and then call them from his own room. You know, people never look at the phone; they just put it to their ear and start talking!

"Most of my friends have passed away now, so it's not as much fun as it used to be. I can sit and talk to the nurses and the respiratory therapists, though. Being in the hospital used to be like going to CF camp; it was so much fun. I miss camp so much! I remember during warm fuzzies one year Rick Zepeda threw copper dust into the closing campfire and it turned green. Camp Ravenswood's cabins left a lot to be desired but that was one of the best camps we had. It was set up perfectly at the very top of the hill with the flagpole. There were a couple of years in a row when we had a dance around the closing campfire. That was perfect, awesome. It almost seems like the end of interaction among cystics now because camp was not only a place to have fun, but you could also learn more about CF there, too. I learned about different stages of my disease and how to cope with it by watching others. It also gave us a chance to get to know other kids who have CF in a nonhospital setting. Now, without camp, it's like the end of a family.

"I'm going to go to school to become a respiratory therapist. Having CF has a lot to do with that. I want to be in a profession in which I can help others who have CF. Being a cystic myself, I think I can be more understanding about their needs and feelings. A lot of the respiratory therapists here at the hospital have become friends with their patients. I think that's what I would do. I could not only be a respiratory therapist, but also at the same time, probably a little bit of an emotional therapist to help cystics cope. Just be there if they need someone to talk to because that's a nice thing to have.

"I was talking on the phone to this guy while I was here in the hospital. He said, 'You know what I don't understand about you? You're always so happy. You've had so many bad cards dealt to your hand, but you always look on the bright side of things.' If I wanted to, I could sit around and feel sorry for myself and say, 'Oh, feel sorry for me; I'm going to die.' But that is not the way to live. That's not living; that's preventing life. I live. I live well."

After a long fight, Jennifer died on July 26, 2001, of a ruptured bowel caused by a bowel obstruction. "I will fight it every inch of the way! I am too stubborn to die," Jennifer often said. She was 26.

OFF TO CF CAMP!

It is not unusual to hear people say that, even though many years have passed, they are still great friends with kids they met at summer camp as a child. CF camp is no different, except the long-term friendships are often replaced with bittersweet memories. Certainly Jennifer was correct about CF camp being lots of fun. It was a time when kids who had CF could get together and be "normal" for a week. Those who didn't have CF (such as siblings, counselors, volunteers, and medical staff) were the ones who were in the minority. CF camp was a time to share stories, talk about life and death, and, like kids everywhere, just hang out and have fun.

> "For an entire week, I was 'normal.' I wasn't 'that girl who coughs a lot' or 'that girl who is always taking medication.' Everybody was just like me, and no one looked at me funny when it came time to do a breathing treatment. Some of my fondest memories are those from CF camp."—Jackie Goryl, 23, a college student from Sterling Heights, Michigan

> "I loved camp because everyone knew what you had. You did not have to explain anything to anyone. Yeah, I think that was the best time. When I tell my friends now that I went to CF camp they're like, 'What is that?' I explain and I'll be like, 'I had the best time of my life.' It was the best experience. I have stories to tell! Sometimes we would stay up all night! I remember once we carried our mattresses from our bunk beds

down this huge hill. We put the mattresses in the middle of the hill, then we'd run and jump on them and slide down. I remember doing that for like two hours in the middle of the night till about five o'clock in the morning! It was me, Nicky, Angela, and I think Jennifer Cherry. I liked when we'd go out sailing or canoeing or boating. The last night with the campfire we would all stay up late and just hang around and talk. I think it was a good experience because I met people. Even though I may not have kept in touch with everyone after camp, I still considered them my friends because when I was with them I felt comfortable; I liked them, I had a good time."—Kimberlee Pilarczyk, in an interview less than a year before she died

◎

"I have several friends who have CF, most of whom I met at CF camp. My relationships are slightly different with them because we can talk about CF-related things without feeling apprehensive or afraid of what they might think. It's fun, in a way, to share experiences and share the good and bad times. Some of my best memories are of times spent with my friends who have CF, mostly during my teens years, when trying to fit in is tough."—Leah K., 22, Orion, Michigan

◎

"I would say my friends with CF are the only friends I have who really understand me and what I have been through and will continue to go through. They are my true peers. I would say there is a different kind of closeness or bond. I feel they were essential to getting me through my teens. CF camp was the only place I felt truly normal as a kid. I feel the benefits far outweigh the risks."—Janelle Benitez, 25, Wisconsin

◎

"I didn't know there was such a thing as CF camp. That's a wonderful idea! When I was a child I was all alone. I lived in Indiana and the other kids were quite cruel. I would have loved to go to a camp where there were other children like me."
—Jessica Hawk-Manus, 25, Nashville, Tennessee

Although uncommon, the memories of camp are less than positive for some. Melissa Kick, a generally "healthier" cystic, comments that camp was "depressing." She says:

"It was so hard to return every year and find out that this friend or that friend had died. It was hard because we were never told the details, the how and why. We would find out when we'd watch the slide show of photos from the year before and realize someone's pictures were missing. Then we'd realize that another friend had died of the same disease we all had. The issue should have been addressed, but the people who ran our camp didn't think they should acknowledge it. That made it especially hard, I think."—Melissa Kick, 26, Libertyville, Illinois

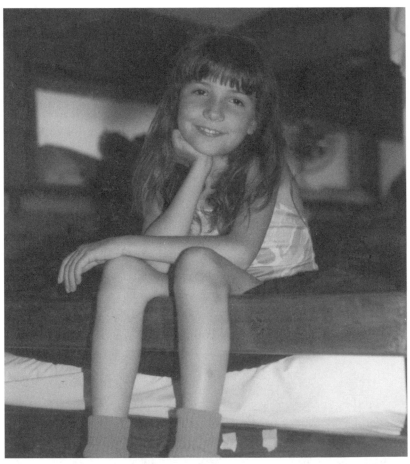

Jackie Goryl waiting to go swimming at CF camp "Onkoi Benek" in Battle Creek, Michigan, 1990.

Unfortunately, because of infection control reasons, doctors began to see CF camps as germ-spreading petri dishes. There are few CF camps in the United States today.

THE PEOPLE I'VE MET

One of the things that I have heard from people who know kids and young adults who have CF is that they are such amazing people. I would have to agree 100 percent.

Closing Campfire

I close my eyes
rest my head.
behind my lids
in the black abyss of
my brain
memories whirl
taking me back
to other weeks
in other years.
They were there
then.
But they are here
now
too
—As surely you understand—
in the stars and
the music and
the pictures and
in that place reserved
in my heart and yours
for them, permanently.
Tears and sweat mingle as we
entwine to console the ache
the longing for that which is lost . . .
Bug repellant permeates the air
Dew covers the grass,
And the sun will shine
On our faces
Our lives
For having been here
And knowing each other.
—Melanie Ann Apel, August 11, 1990

Because they spend so much time in the hospital and around adults, many children who have CF possess a certain maturity that their healthier peers do not have. They are able to talk to adults and children in matter-of-fact tones. And it's not uncommon to hear how someone with CF has positively—and sometimes profoundly—affected the lives of those who had the privilege of knowing them. Of course, this goes both ways, and those who have CF have positive things to say about the people they know because of their illness.

"The best thing about having CF is the people I've met and the friends I've made. The hospital is a whole second home to me. One of the kids I know from the hospital is a boy named Devon. He's 15 and I've known him forever. We've grown up together at the hospital. He's made a real impact on me. He's gotten sicker in the past few years. He's on oxygen now. And then there's Katie Kocelko. She's had two double lung transplants. It's amazing. She's amazing! She came home for the weekend from St. Louis, where she'd just had her second transplant, so she could go to prom!"—Maggie Sheehan, 15

Of course, sometimes there's a downside to meeting such wonderful people. Sometimes they die. But, as Maggie Sheehan sees it, there's still always something good to be experienced and something to learn.

"Kristine was a longtime friend of mine at Children's Memorial. I met her through Jennifer Cherry during one of our admissions. She was almost 20 years older than I am, so she was friends with my mom, too. She was treated at Children's Memorial until she was 28, then she transferred to the adult CF center at Northwestern. She was someone to look up to. I looked at her to see the things I might do when I'm older. Well, she was on the transplant list for new lungs. But things kept happening that prevented her from getting them. I knew she was sick, but I didn't know how sick. It didn't surprise me a lot when she died. She's the first person I was close to who died. It wasn't as bad as I thought it would be. I don't see dying as a real tragedy. I'm sad that she's gone, but she's in a better place than here. I'll see her later on. It's better than suffering. She suffered a lot."—Maggie Sheehan

HOW OLD IS HE?! REALLY BEATING THE ODDS

Perhaps one of the most interesting and inspirational stories illustrating someone actually living a "normal life" despite cystic fibrosis comes out of Norwich, Connecticut. Harold A. Soloff, JD, MS, associate, University of London, attorney-at-law (retired), Hal to his friends and family, was born with cystic fibrosis before cystic fibrosis officially "existed." Now 72 years old, Hal shares his story.

"I was born in 1931," Hal begins his amazing tale. "As a baby, I had experienced bowel blockage and was treated with things like castor oil and milk of magnesia. CF wasn't 'invented' until I was 7 years old. That was 1938. My lung functioning was good until 1939 when I was 8, and, due to the heat (we lived in Dallas at the time), I spent the whole summer in the hospital on IVs. My sister was born with cystic fibrosis that year. I had a brother who was three years younger, but he died soon after being born. My sister married at age 18 and at age 19 became pregnant. Her CF doctor advised her to terminate the pregnancy due to her ill health. She refused and died at age 20, six weeks after bearing a baby girl. The baby girl is now married and has two brilliant and beautiful young ladies of her own.

"When I was a child, cystic fibrosis was unknown. I was treated by excellent doctors for the symptoms. Obviously, they knew what they were doing. CF has always forced choices in my life, and I have gone with the flow, including a career change and many postponements of planned trips and other activities when I'm not feeling well enough to go.

"I was diagnosed at Boston Children's Hospital when I was 28 years old. I have *pseudomonas*, *Staph A* and aspergillus colonies in my lungs and sinuses. My first major sign of CF was continuous sinus infections from my early teens, necessitating major surgeries and subsequent polypoid tissue removals through the years. While visiting my childhood ENT specialist in Boston (I was born in Connecticut), he suggested that I be tested for CF. The sweat tests proved positive. I have since had voluntary investigative surgery and two DNA studies.

"I was an attorney and stockbroker at the time, and I had been married for three years. The doctors thought my health was poor and advised, at the rate I was going, I could expect perhaps three or so more years to live. My wife, a teacher, convinced me to go back to grad school, get a masters degree, and teach. I did and taught for twenty-five more years.

"I have GERD (gastro-esophageal reflux disease) for which I take Prevacid, and mild digestive factors, which require the use of enzymes. I have suffered several bouts of hemoptysis (coughing up blood). I take Zithromax as a prophylactic antibiotic and various antibiotics when there are flare-ups. Fortunately, I have not needed an IV for several years. Due to the aging process (yeah!), I take other medications for mild high blood pressure, osteoarthritis, and so forth, and I have hypoglycemia, which requires that I not eat sugar and restrict my diet.

"My medical record looks something like this: digestive and bowel problems: infancy; lung dysfunction: hospitalized at age 8; sinus infections: age 12; sinus surgeries: age 15, 17, 18, and major subsequent polypoid tissue removals through the years; began regimen of antibiotics and inhalation machine treatments for lung and sinus infections: age 15 in 1946 (I recently was interviewed and put on the Pfizer web page for taking their antibiotics since 1946); GERD: age 42; and first major hemoptysis: age 44 while living in London, UK, [where] I was hospitalized and received excellent treatment. When infections in my lungs and sinuses appear to be getting the upper hand, I use my mini inhalation machine with either an antibiotic or DNAse (which is not very effective with me), plus oral antibiotics. IVs usually have not been necessary, but I have used them. I am presently taking Zithromax, Levaquin, and Sporonox (for the aspergillus).

"CF is insidious and attacks different people in different ways. If one lives long enough, one can expect to enjoy the aches and pains of the aging process. Sob . . . lost my hair! Exercise and sticking to their medication regimen will help!"

Hal has outlived the median age of those who have CF by decades. What is his secret?

"Never lying to my mother," Hal says, "and I listen to my body and am disciplined to follow the regimen necessary for survival. I have always fought hard to reach my goals and have maintained a sense of humor. I've had excellent medical care, love and care from my wife, and support from our children, family, and friends. I was very physically active as a child even though I was short and underweight. I began taking drum lessons at age 10 and marched in the primary school band. I was on the boxing team in high school and fought in the Golden Gloves. I played in the marching band and the orchestra. I went to the Julliard School of Music in New York at age 17 and studied percussion (precollege program), and I attended Northwestern University and marched in the band there. I was offered scholarships to six universities due to my music abilities. I continued as a professional percussionist (symphony, opera, and dance combo) until I went to law school. I still have my drums and blast away with my favorite bands' CDs."—Harold Soloff

WHEN I'M NOT TAKING A TREATMENT

With daily nebulizers and bronchial drainage regimens, medicine cabinets full of pills, and enzymes for digestion of every meal, it is a wonder anyone who has CF can get anything else accomplished in a day. Oh, but how those who live with CF make the most of their days, including planning for the future.

"Spare time? What's that? (Just kidding!) I like to do fairly normal things, I guess: listening to and playing a bit of music, reading, doing various things on the computer (some programming, web design, surfing the Internet), talking to friends, playing video games, watching TV and movies, and a dwindling few good shows on U.S. television (no more reality shows, please!). I also enjoy cooking from time to time (cleaning up is much less enjoyable, sadly), biking, boating (Guntersville has a large lake and we recently bought a boat), driving around, and so on. Of course, I do chores (dishes, cleaning the kitchen, mowing the lawn, taking out the trash, etc.) as well, but those obviously aren't quite as much fun."
—James Lawlor, 17, Guntersville, Alabama

"In a perfect world, I want a family. More than anything, I want to have a husband and children of my own. My career is important to me, but ultimately, I want to have a family. I am working toward a bachelor's degree in occupational therapy, which is a great field for me. I have unending empathy for what patients go through, as my CF has helped me to understand and acknowledge even the smallest effects that an illness or accident can have on a person. I might even consider graduate school, but that depends on my health. Since this is obviously not a perfect world, I don't know what will happen. I will certainly have my career, as I am close to finishing my schooling. I see myself with a husband, but I am not so sure about having children. It depends on my health and the possibility of the

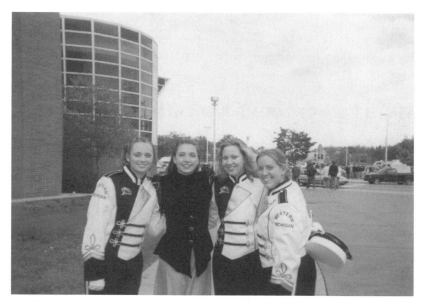

Game Day, October 2001. Jackie Goryl, second from left, and fellow high school band members.

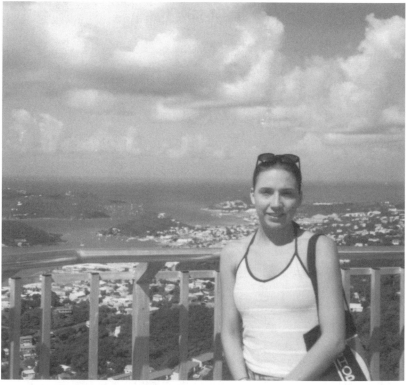

In May 2003 Jackie Goryl and her mother went on a pregraduation vacation—a Caribbean cruise! This is Jackie in St. Thomas.

child having CF. It is hard for me to knowingly take the risk of having a child with CF (if my husband turns out to be a carrier) after knowing what I, and others with the disease, have experienced. I also want to travel. I want to see some of Europe—Germany or Italy, anything!"—Jackie Goryl, 23

⊚

"Ideally I would like to get married when I'm 23. I would probably qualify as a chartered accountant, but I'm not sure if I'll be able to cope with working for a firm of chartered accountants. Luckily, I'll be able to work from home if I want to or maybe at a tertiary institution, which would mean a lot of holidays."—Alice Vosloo, 19

⊚

"My plans for the immediate future are to get a nursing job right after I graduate and to eventually pursue my career in another state. I may even go back to college eventually to further my degree. I would absolutely love to get married to a wonderful man and have children if my health permits. But regardless of my ability to have children, I want to adopt, as well. I don't feel that there should be anything holding me back from my dreams and ambitions because I have a lot of plans ahead."—Leah K., 22, Orion, Michigan

⊚

"I love to work out, swim, and bowl if my strength permits it. I enjoy cross-stitching, cooking, the Internet, staying in touch with other CF people, and going to the movies." —Jessica Hawk-Manus

Did You Know? American Airlines is corporate partner of the Cystic Fibrosis Foundation, and Interstate Hotels and Resorts is a Cystic Fibrosis Foundation national sponsor.[1]

A SICK SENSE OF HUMOR

Have you ever heard someone say that laughter is the best medicine? If you have known someone who has CF, one thing you will remember is his or her laugh, usually in direct response to his or her wacky sense of humor. After all, if you can find humor in a situation, no matter how bad it is, things will not look quite so desperate.

Wendy and her dad Mitch have the perfect example of a classic CF sense of humor:

> "I thought my family and I were crazy, but I guess not. I'm not sure exactly how we came to call it this, but we called those big green mucus plugs I used to cough up 'yum-yums.' It was my dad's idea—[he has a] rather warped sense of humor that I also inherited! Then one day we saw a place called 'Yum Yum Yogurt' and my parents and I cracked up!"—Wendy Abrams, 21, Miami, Florida

◎

> "My son, Joe, and I always yell, 'Loogie flying' when we spit out the window or are walking across the parking lot. Yuk!" —Christie Rodecap, Fort Wayne, Indiana

◎

> "Sometimes I would take the slimy, greenish colored silly putty and put it in my hand without anyone noticing. Then I'd sneeze or cough into the hand and show the silly putty and disgust everyone in the room. That one always got some gags!" —Jennie Gibson, 26, Redmond, Washington, had a double lung transplant on November 21, 2001

Or what about the woman who says a friend of hers once referred to her mucus as guacamole? Pass the chips! Even the littlest kids with CF come up with some amusing ways to describe their mucus. "Betsy, my four-year-old daughter who has CF, has been calling her mucus 'pickles' since she was two," says Mary Sullivan of San Antonio, Texas. "She'll cough and say, 'I just have some pickles in my lungs.' She calls her enzymes 'birdseed' because we still open the capsules and sprinkle them. It's very cute. It would be a lot cuter if she didn't have CF, but oh well."

On occasion, the humor might not be classified as "sick," but again it comes as an illustration of the importance of seeing the funny side of otherwise serious situations.

"We purchased a new neb compressor for our daughter last summer. It was used without incident that evening. The next day, when we turned it on for her morning treatment, it made an odd rattling sound. Upon closer inspection, I could see a nickel stuck in one of the vented slots and a quarter on the floor of the compressor casing. It seems Stefany's* little brother Saul*, who was 4 years old at the time, mistook the neb compressor for a new-fangled piggy bank!"—Molly Jansen*, Huntersville, North Carolina, mom of Stefany*, 15

Diane Meyer, a respiratory therapist at Chicago's Children's Memorial Hospital, remembers well the sense of humor of one very special patient:

"It couldn't have been more than two or three days before Angela died," Diane begins, referring to 19-year-old Angela Dibbern, who lost her battle with cystic fibrosis in 1987. "She was really short of breath then. I couldn't believe she was trying to be funny, yet she was laughing. She had the TV on in the background and Gorbachev was getting off a plane coming to

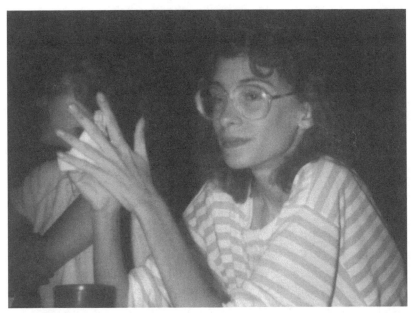

Angela Dibbern at CF camp in 1987 just a few months before she died at age 19. Soft-spoken Angela was a most impressive young lady. She was enrolled in college, earned high grades, worked part time, and battled CF with a full-scale sense of humor.

visit the United States. They started playing the Soviet national anthem. She was waving her hand, pulling me down. I said, 'What's the matter?' She said, 'It sounds like the Bozo theme song!'"

BUT SOMETIMES THERE IS ANGER

Most people who have cystic fibrosis handle their situations with humor and dignity; yet, there are times when, despite all efforts, anger rises to the surface and takes over. The anger might be directed at the disease. The anger might be directed toward those who don't have CF, such as siblings, friends, or the general population. Anger might be aimed at family members, at doctors who can't prescribe a cure, at fate for the way things turned out, and sometimes even at God. Or your anger might not be for yourself but for someone else—a friend, a child, a sibling—who gets sick and dies. You feel it's unfair that someone you love has to be in pain and suffer! You might even be angry at cystic fibrosis itself. Sometimes it just seems as if you just can't catch a break with this disease. Anger comes as no surprise when you consider the ramifications of cystic fibrosis. After all, this is a life-threatening disease.

Anger can strike at any time, whether you're the person who has CF or the person who loves someone who has CF. There are as many ways to deal with your anger as there are reasons to be angry. Some people throw things, others take out their aggression on the field of their favorite sport, still others write about their feelings in a journal, and some seek therapy from an outside source, such as a counselor, social worker, therapist, or support group. If you are having trouble managing your anger, consider speaking to a nurse or doctor at your CF clinic. He or she should be able to direct you toward help.

Whether you are a teen who has CF, a friend or sibling of someone who has CF, or a parent reading this book because you have a child of your own who has CF, the anger you experience is real, and it is shared by many others in your situation.

"I have gotten angry so many times at CF. My teen years were the hardest because I was really sick. I had to be evaluated for transplant at age 15. There were times when I got mad at my parents because obviously they are the reason why I was born with this disease. I only felt anger from time to time and it always passed, and then I would be fine. The anger never lasted. But when I was angry, I would do anything bad that I'm not supposed to do like, believe it or not, I used to smoke cigarettes. Yuck! I think, though, that CF turned out to be a real blessing to me because it has made me strong and it's the reason why I'm the person that I am."
—April Harris-Kinsey, 20, Englewood, Florida

You can lobby your state senators to make May the National Cystic Fibrosis Awareness Month. For more information, please visit www.ncfac.org.

"How could you *not* get angry?" begins Val, whose granddaughter Tara Ann Daily has cystic fibrosis. "First you get angry at God. Then you get angry at your friends with healthy children, your spouse for donating half of the genes, the universe for continuing to function when your whole life has been turned upside down . . . and finally, at yourself because whether you are a parent or grandparent you did contribute the genes. But those are all parts of the grief process; I was able to get over that, and within a few weeks I understood that some things just are! There is no blame. There is no shame. There should be no jealousy. What there should be is anger at the disease and frustration at our inability to do enough to make our loved ones not sick anymore. And there should also be a gratefulness for the blessings that have been brought into our lives: for this unbelievably special person; for the people who have come into our lives while we face the challenges this horrible disease inflicts on the whole family; and for the

increase in our faith as it is challenged time and again (do we really turn to God when in desperation? Yeah!). Is there a medicine right around the corner that will effect a cure and will save Tara from all of this? We certainly hope and pray so, but people who have CF say they have been hearing this for fifteen years. So, in the meantime, we plan for the worst, pray and hope for the best, and deal with what we get. However, we remain very, very angry. You have to in order to deal with it and to have the will to kick CF butt!"
—Val Phillips, Naples, Texas

> **As I lay me down to sleep and say a little prayer**
> **I can't help but shed a tear for all these years**
> **they've been telling us a CF cure is near**
> **All our little angels—flying, flying away**
> **Oh God, why can't there be a cure *today***
> **Your precious gifts You have given us—smile,**
> **laugh, and love**
> **Their call to heaven is much too soon as they**
> **journey to above**
> **I will dream of the breath of life—for one, for**
> **all, for us**
> **Lord thank you for giving me this chance to say**
> **And giving me another day**
> **—Heidi Kirschbaum, mother of Heather, 12**

"Being 16, I'm just at the end stage of the horrific teen years, as my dad likes to put it. He thinks I'm slowly getting better every day. I was a vicious little teen. Yes, I do get angry at times, generally when I find myself restricted from doing something and realizing this is primarily due to this disease. I have a lot of stress in my life for a teen. My ambition to do well is killing me. I want to combat this disease and just prove to myself and everyone else that I can do it even though I have this disease. My ambition was law: to do extremely well in my end-of-school state exams and go to college to study law. I shattered my own dream. I realized I miss so much school due to CF, on average a day a week. I'm too tired and I get sick easily, and I can't keep up with the pace of an able-bodied person. I figured even if I graduate with an honors law degree and become a

lawyer, who wants to hire a representative that may not be able to be in full attendance because of illness? Answer: nobody. I don't know how I deal with my anger; I don't. I've lost faith in myself, and I just don't have a clue what I want to do now when I leave school or what to do in college. When I become so angry I hate myself, I hate my body, I hate my genes, and unfortunately (I hate myself for this one), I do get very angry at my parents. They created me and I'm the one suffering. The usual selfish question used to float around everywhere: Why me? I've accepted a lot more in the last eighteen months, and I've learned that nothing is going to make this disease go away. It's a part of me and I've got to get on with it. It has actually made me as a person, too. Without CF I wouldn't have half the memories I have, both good and bad. I wouldn't be who I am today without CF; I'd be someone else with perfect genes."
—Faela Smyth, 16, Dublin, Ireland

Marge is the mother of three gorgeous daughters, Angela, April, and Candice. Candice, 22, is the youngest. April, 23, does not have CF. Angela was 25 years old when she died of CF complications on October 28, 2003. Marge says:

"I think pretty much for everyone the anger is directed at the disease itself and never for the person you love. The anger can pop up because you feel helpless and can't control or stop the progression of the disease—maybe from stress, too, being tired and overwhelmed. I think in their teen years my girls more or less resented that they couldn't be 'normal' like everyone else, and they got rebellious with having to take medicines and do therapies. Both Angela and Candice took their turn at trying to ignore the fact that they had CF. They both figured they were going to die anyway, so why not enjoy life. This only lasted for short periods off and on. Angela's major anger was directed toward the medical professionals and the disease itself. Anger often comes into play when you're dealing with hospitals and a lot of the idiots out there who are totally oblivious to what you're going through. Right now my anger is directed at the carelessness of hospitals and doctors, as well as their 'God complex.'"—Marge Budnieski, Mokena, Illinois

121

Marie is the mother of Rachel, 21, who has CF, CFRD, and has recently undergone a double lung transplant:

"Angry? Never! And I am such a liar. How do you handle anger at something you can't scream at, hit, or accuse? It is like punching a wave that knocks you over in the ocean. Praying, ranting to people who love us and share our frustration, and talking to others who understand [all help]. But the divorce rate is high [for parents of kids who have CF]; perhaps this is part of it."
—Marie Dexter

Did You Know?
Football great Boomer Esiason's son, Gunnar, has cystic fibrosis. Since Gunnar's diagnosis in 1993, Boomer and his wife, Cheryl, have worked to support the search for a cure for CF. You can visit Boomer's CF website at www.esiason.org.

Some use sports to vent their anger, as does 14-year-old Ben Monaco. About Ben's anger management, his mother Marcia says:

"He gets angry about having to do all of his treatments when his friends are doing what they want. He also gets angry that he has to deal with the stigma that goes with the learning delays he suffered from the severe infection and illness he had when he was 2 years old. One thing he does that helps manage his anger is Tai Kwon Do. When Ben first started Tai Kwon Do, it was because I had read that it was good to help in airway clearance and lung strengthening for kids with CF. He has been taking it for about three and a half years, and he became a black belt on March 28, 2004. It has been great for him. He can get so angry, ranting and complaining; then it is time to go to his Tai Kwon Do class. He comes home a different kid. He gets such a workout and lets out all of that pent up energy. It really seems to help."—Marcia Monaco, Columbus, Ohio

Some people, like Rebecca, take a more philosophical look at the problem:

"CF is like a lens through which I see and thus interpret the world. The priorities of our culture, like independence, absolute autonomy, and workaholism before health, anger me in reference to CF or any chronic illness. I feel that with enough time and support I can stay well and really contribute to society, and in my experience, people have been more than happy to help. However, I harbor the desire to be totally independent, to not ask for help, and to plan my life around my disease so that I never need help or so that I can pay for help (i.e., if I am sick) so that my disease does not trouble others, and I think that this is very much a part of the American self-help ethos. Sometimes I feel like making a declaration of *dependence* as it would make my life so much easier. I certainly wish I could depend on someone other than my employer for health insurance and that the government offered more help paying for medicine and health care.

"How do I deal with anger regarding these things; how do I deal with CF? I study. In college I studied medicine and health from the social sciences; now I study diabetes as a research coordinator at the University Hospital. I hope to become a medical anthropologist so that I can study our culture in reference to illness and people who are chronically ill. For me, it is hard to get angry about CF because there is no one to direct the anger at. Anger is most productive when it is directed at the people and things that one might be able to affect or change. So I am more likely to get angry that CF doctors failed to tell me something or that my illness was such a financial burden on my parents, as these are things we can and should work to change. As for being mad about having CF, anger wells up and boils over almost exclusively when I am feeling *really* run down, perhaps too run down to funnel it toward a productive end, or when I am on prednisone. In case of the latter, I kid you not,

---

ANOTHER BOOK WORTH READING

Alive at 25 (Atlanta: Longstreet Press, 2002) by Andy Lipman is an inspirational look at overcoming obstacles and living life in the face of adversity. Andy Lipman writes about how he beat the odds of cystic fibrosis. You can visit Andy's website at www.aliveat25.org.

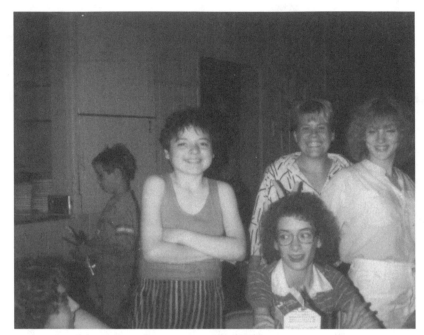

These are five of the girls from my 1986 CF camp cabin (from left to right): Cris Shadle (in the bottom left corner), Lisa Zepeda, Angela Dibbern, Jenny Morrison, and Fonda Langston. Jenny (with the short hair and making "bunny ears") is the only survivor of the group. Now in her mid-30s, Jenny is the only one who has reached and surpassed the median age for CF. In addition, she gave birth to a healthy daugher, who is now a teen herself.

throwing things and pulling my hair and yelling usually help. My mother even offered to pick up some thrift store dishes and volunteered the outdoor brick wall for smashing them. I don't know exactly how I dealt with anger as a teen, as is the case now, I wasn't all that angry about CF."—Rebecca Mueller, 22, Philadelphia

Feeling angry is part of the natural process of dealing with a life-threatening disease. Facing your anger takes a great deal of strength and courage.

NOTE

1. Cystic Fibrosis Foundation, cff.org/about_cf/what_is_cf.cfm? CFID=1619012&CFTOKEN=84991526.

Other Complications

7

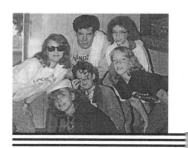

Although people who have CF are living longer lives today because of better treatments, in an unfortunate catch-22, their quality of life might actually be at risk as they get older. The Cystic Fibrosis Foundation's website states the following: "Adults may experience additional health challenges including CF-related diabetes and osteoporosis."

> **The Cystic Fibrosis Foundation was established in 1955 for the purpose of finding new treatments and a cure for cystic fibrosis.**

In addition to having cystic fibrosis, two of the campers, Lisa and Josè, had another illness to contend with. They had diabetes. What a drag, I thought, as if CF weren't enough. What I didn't realize at the time—what I think many of us didn't realize—was that diabetes was not just a random cruelty bestowed upon these kids. As I would later learn, diabetes is just one of many CF-related complications that is likely to crop up for many of the kids and young adults who have CF if they are lucky to live long enough. When it comes to cystic fibrosis, it would seem, the gift of longevity is not without charge. As if having CF weren't enough.

The list of complications related to cystic fibrosis can be divided into two categories. The first would be a list of complications that one would expect to find in just about anyone who has cystic fibrosis (at one time or another) and are due to CF itself. This list would be comprised of things like:

- Nasal polyps
- Sinusitis
- *Pseudomonas aeruginosa*
- *Burkholderia cepacia*
- Hemoptysis

The second list would be comprised of complications that set in when a person who has cystic fibrosis lives longer than expected and the damage done by CF and the medications used to fight it begin to take their toll on the body. This list would include:

- Arthritis
- Osteoporosis
- Diabetes
- MRSA
- Liver disease

Let's look at some of these, beginning with the first list:

THE NOSE: NASAL POLYPS AND SINUSITIS

Ten to 20 percent of people who have CF experience nasal polyps, which frequently require surgery to remove. Nasal polyps are "small protrusions of tissue from the lining of the nose that go into the nasal cavity." In addition to the polyps, it is common for people who have CF to have recurring sinus infections.[1]

Sinusitis is simply an inflammation of the nasal sinuses.

PSEUDOMONAS AERUGINOSA AND *BURKHOLDERIA CEPACIA*

You've already read about *Pseudomonas aeruginosa* in chapter 1.

In the early 1990s, a new threat to the lives of those who have CF came onto the battleground. *Burkholderia cepacia* (*B. cepacia*) is a bacterium that is resistant to most available drugs. It is spread from person to person or from object to person. Only a few antibiotics have any effect on *B. cepacia*, which makes catching it something that people who have CF do not want to do. Once a person who has CF contracts B. *cepacia*, he or she will be unable to get rid of the bug. Like other bacteria, *B. cepacia* will take residence in the lungs as a permanent infection, destroying healthy lung tissue and, like *pseudomonas* before it, *B. cepacia* hastens death.

B. cepacia, known to most people who have CF as simply "cepacia," does not have any impact on people who are healthy, such as caregivers for those who have CF. *Cepacia* is routinely tested for during sputum culture. Good hand washing and proper hygiene, such as covering mouth and nose when coughing, using a tissue, and cleaning up after coughing, are the best ways to prevent transmission of *cepacia* from one patient to another via healthcare workers. But sadly, the best way to

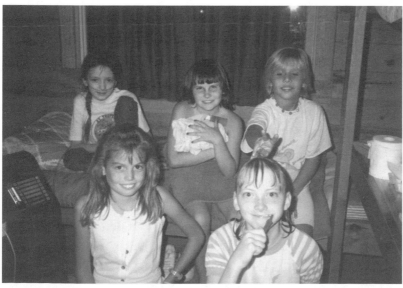

I dragged these 10-year-old girls out of our cabin bathroom for this photo. Elyce (top left) was on oxygen almost continuously. She died before Christmas that year (1988). Of the other four—Angela, Melissa, Kerri, and Amy—both Melissa (making "rabbit ears") and Kerri (bottom left) are in their late 20s now. Kerri works as a neonatal nurse and has just gotten married.

prevent the transmission of *cepacia* among those who have CF is to ban contact between those who have *cepacia* and those who do not. This is in stark contrast to the trend years ago to get people who have CF together so that they could socialize with others in common.[2] Thank goodness for email! It is because of the threat of *cepacia* that many CF camps have ceased.

Many hospitals no longer allow cystic fibrosis patients to room with one another for fear of spreading germs such as *cepacia*. In fact, some hospitals no longer even allow CF patients to have face-to-face contact with each other. When contact is unavoidable, such as while waiting in a CF clinic waiting room, patients are asked to wear surgical masks over their mouth and nose.

> "I hate the isolation now. Whenever I am in the hospital, I have to put on a mask if I am going to be in contact with others who have CF. I don't have *cepacia*. I know the mask is to protect me from others who do have it. But that mask makes me feel alone, as if I were already dead."—Chad Lucci, 25, Boulder, Colorado

HEMOPTYSIS

Hemoptysis sounds like some sort of very large prehistoric beast. As in, "Let's learn about T-rex and his pal Hemoptysis today." Actually, hemoptysis is just a fancy medical term that means "coughing up blood." For some people who have cystic fibrosis, coughing up blood is a regular occurrence. For others who do not experience hemoptysis regularly, the first time it happens is terribly frightening. Because of chronic infection in the lungs, damage occurs. Sometimes this damage manifests itself in the form of broken blood vessels. When this happens, along with mucus, blood will come forth during an episode of coughing.

> "When I was a freshman in high school, they tried fixing the bleeding by going through my femoral vein and using polyethylene tubing to advance up into my pulmonary artery.

Then they injected some dye so they could see all the arteries and the areas that were bleeding. My lungs were bleeding because of so much infection and because of eroded vessels. They saw on the X-ray where the arteries and veins were affected. Then they injected a solution that cauterized the area. It was very painful; I remember it! I wasn't supposed to know what was going on. I asked and asked to be put to sleep, but they had to keep me conscious so they would not suppress my respiratory rate. I remember everything! That was the only way of helping the problem, but it didn't stop it from occurring again in other areas of my lungs. I had it done just that one time and I wouldn't do it again. I told my mom I'd die bleeding before I'd ever do it again because it hurt so much. They couldn't do my other lung anyway. The bleeding was too close to the jugular vein, and they didn't want to embolize that area.

"My biggest problem was coughing up blood. It would come whenever it felt like it. I could be lying in bed or I could be walking in school; it didn't matter. I had maybe thirty seconds to when I knew it was coming. It felt like leaking. I could feel it leaking into my lung, kind of like breathing under water. I knew what it was. It was different from the rattle of the mucus. It's a lot more like water. I would only have so much time to get to the bathroom before the blood would come. It would last five or ten minutes. I was becoming anemic because I was losing so much blood. I was tired of that. I was tired of having to worry about where I was going to be when the blood came.

"And that's what it's like to cough up blood."—Amy Thom, 19

DIABETES

"Supposedly I had CF-related diabetes, or CFRD for short. But it turned out I didn't. It was right around my birthday last year, when I went in for my yearly checkup. My blood sugar was really high, so I was instructed to test my blood sugar four times a day. And I had to see a specialist. This was really discouraging for me. It was just one more layer to deal with on top of everything else I go through on a daily basis. I was pretty depressed after this diagnosis. Then it turned out I didn't have

CFRD after all. Well, not for now, anyway. I will eventually. Even though I have already been through this experience, I don't think I will deal with this very well when it happens for real. But you can't ignore diabetes. Fortunately now they have a new forearm stick, which is easier than sticking your finger to get blood. I put IVs in people every day at work, so I think I can give myself a shot of insulin if I have to."—Chad Lucci

"I was diagnosed with borderline diabetes when I was 11 and full diabetes when I was 12. They found out when I had a physical done at my pediatrician's office. They tested my blood sugar and it was high so then they made me get further testing done, and there, sure enough, I had diabetes. That's when the shots started. It wasn't too hard learning to do the shots. They had a nurse come to my house daily to give me my shots until I could do it myself, after about a week. I handled it the way I've handled everything else in my life: learn to master it, and move on!"—April Harris-Kinsey, 20, Englewood, Florida

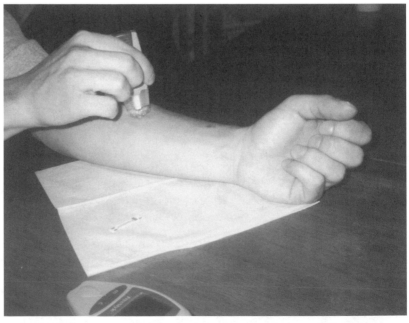

Those with CFRD must regularly test their blood sugar. This little gizmo makes a small prick in the skin, drawing blood.

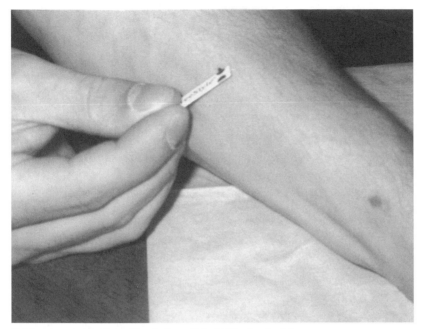

A blood sample is collected on this little test strip.

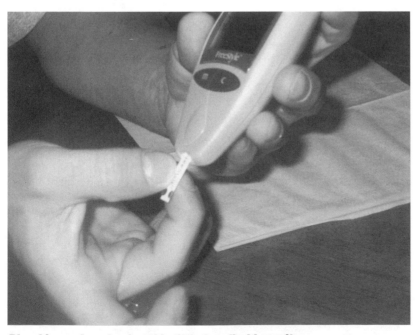

Blood is analyzed using this little handheld monitor.

Diabetes is a serious disease unto itself. Like cystic fibrosis, there is no cure for diabetes. But there are treatments that, if followed properly, can greatly enhance the lives of those who have diabetes. You already know that the pancreas is responsible for producing the enzymes necessary for the digestion of food and that this system is generally impaired in a person who has CF. The pancreas is also in charge of producing a hormone called insulin. Insulin is necessary to control the levels of blood sugar, also known as glucose, in the body. When the pancreas does not produce enough insulin, a person becomes diabetic. Without the necessary insulin, glucose levels rise, and the person gets very sick. There are several different types of diabetes, the most common of which are called insulin-dependent diabetes mellitus, or IDDM, and non-insulin-dependent diabetes mellitus, or NIDDM. A person who has IDDM must take insulin shots to provide his or her body with the necessary insulin, as the body's white blood cells destroy all the insulin-secreting cells in the pancreas. A person who has NIDDM can often be treated with diet or other medications. CF-related diabetes, or CFRD, is similar to both IDDM and NIDDM but is not specifically either one. The term CFRD encompasses a variety of different diabetic conditions. Some people who have CF-related diabetes must always take insulin, others only need insulin on occasion, and still others only have occasional, random abnormalities with their glucose levels.

Because of the thick, sticky mucus produced by the body of the person who as CF, the pancreas becomes not only obstructed but also eventually damaged. Many of the insulin-producing cells are destroyed, leaving the CF young adult with less insulin than normal. If the insulin level drops too low, insulin injections are needed to control the glucose levels, and the person is said to have CF-related diabetes.[3] Any combination of the following can cause diabetes in people who have CF.

⊚ **Insulin deficiency. The pancreas in a person who has CF does not make sufficient insulin because of damage caused by thick, sticky mucus.**

- Insulin resistance. The body does not properly use its insulin, resulting in the need for more insulin to metabolize food.

- Some medications can cause the blood sugar levels to increase, which can eventually lead to diabetes.

- Infection can predispose a person to diabetes.

> "I only have CFRD when I go on steroids, so I really don't do steroids anymore." —Janelle Benitez

Symptoms of CFRD

- Frequent urination
- Excessive thirst
- Excessive fatigue
- Unexplained weight loss[4]

About half of all people who have CFRD need daily insulin injections to keep their glucose levels down. The other half have intermittent CFRD and only need to take insulin on occasion because they still make a small amount of insulin, and their bodies are sensitive enough to the insulin that they maintain normal glucose levels. Certain events such as infection or surgery could cause these people to need insulin injections temporarily.

People who have CF and who show abnormal glucose levels even though they do not have CFRD are said to have a condition known as impaired glucose tolerance. High levels of impaired glucose tolerance indicate a high risk for developing CFRD.

While Chad acknowledges the importance of not ignoring CFRD, for some who have CF, adding a diagnosis of diabetes is simply too much.

"Dietary issues were huge for me when I was a child. Since I was 9 I was told that in order to maintain my weight, I had to eat a high-fat, high-calorie, high-carbohydrate diet. Then to be told that I have CFRD and I have to cut all of those things plus the sugars and the complex carbohydrates but still maintain my weight . . . ! It's really hard to make that change."—Chad Lucci

"I have to keep a regular CF diet despite my diabetes. I just take more insulin to cover the carbohydrates and sugars I take in."—Jessica Hawk-Manus

In order to keep blood sugar levels where they belong, a well-balanced diet is key. Frequent glucose level checks, as well as insulin shots when (or if) needed, will help a person with CFRD stay healthy. Usually a healthful diet consisting of three well-balanced meals and snacks is good enough. Often meals and snacks must be scheduled specifically to meet the body's needs. Insulin doses are often adjusted daily based on blood sugar levels as well as expected carbohydrate intake.[5]

On average, the onset of CFRD occurs in young adults between the ages of 18 and 21, although people have been known to get CFRD at younger and older ages. It is not unusual for someone to have CFRD for a few years without even knowing it. In one study, nearly 30 percent of the people who had CFRD did not experience any symptoms of hyperglycemia (high blood sugar) or unexplained weight loss.[6]

MRSA

The acronym MRSA, which is pronounced "MER-sa," stands for Methicillin Resistant *Staphylococcus aureus (S. aureus)*. Quite a mouthful, which is why it's commonly referred to as simply MRSA.

Methicillin was an antibiotic used to treat *S. aureus* in the early 1960s before it was replaced by less toxic "cousins" such as Flucoxacillin. MRSA is resistant to Flucoxacillin, the most commonly used antibiotic for anti-staphylococcal prophylaxis and treatment of patients with cystic fibrosis (CF). It is also resistant to the cephalosporins. Many strains are also resistant to other common antibiotics such as erythromycin and the quinolones, for example, Ciprofloxacin. The first reported isolation of a methicillin-resistant *S. aureus* occurred in London in 1961.[7]

It is not known just how many people who have CF also have MRSA. It is known that one of the risk factors for colonizing MRSA is staying in the hospital too long.

MRSA is transmitted on hands or on articles such as bedding and can colonize in different parts of the body such as the nose and throat and other moist areas.[8] Studies have shown that while children infected with MRSA do not have significantly worse respiratory function, they may have more stunted growth. Children who have MRSA need significantly more courses of IV antibiotics, and they have a worse chest X-ray than those who do not.[9]

Some people can be colonized with MRSA but not actually be infected with it. A number of those who have MRSA might eventually get rid of it. While it does not appear that MRSA itself causes any serious damage to the lungs, it is often hard to make that judgment accurately as many people who have MRSA also have infections such as *pseudomonas* or *cepacia*.[10]

Eighty percent of children with cystic fibrosis are born to parents with no prior history of the disease.[11]

Both arthritis and osteoporosis are mentioned on this list as well. It just goes to show that CF is not a wholly limited disease. Eventually, either the disease itself or the medications used to combat it will begin to do damage to the entire body if given the chance.

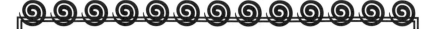

ANOTHER BOOK WORTH READING

In *From a Taste of Salt* (Frederick, MD: PublishAmerica, 2004), Marcella Callicutt writes about the happy times and the sad times that came with being the mother of three daughters, all of whom had cystic fibrosis.

LIVER DISEASE

Like the lungs, the liver is another organ often affected by cystic fibrosis, necessitating a transplant. Unlike the lungs, however, whether or not a person develops liver problems is far more unpredictable than the likelihood that he or she will have lung problems due to CF.

Many people who have CF have absolutely no liver involvement. There is no true predictor of whether or not one will eventually develop liver involvement, although there is some increased likelihood that children born with meconium ileus could have a greater chance of developing liver problems later on. There is also some evidence that boys are more likely to develop liver problems than girls.

The liver disease itself varies greatly from person to person, and the progress varies just as much. Liver damage begins in the small bile ducts. Like other secretions in the body, the bile in these ducts produced by the liver cells is particularly sticky and causes the ducts to become blocked. Similar to the damaging process occurring in the lungs, liver tissue in the surrounding area becomes damaged and scarred. This situation is called biliary fibrosis.

Biliary fibrosis progresses much like CF itself, and eventually the entire liver becomes damaged. The liver actually becomes hard. It becomes difficult for blood to flow through the liver. It ceases to function properly.[12] When damage reaches this stage, a liver transplant becomes necessary to sustain life.

Perhaps a third list of CF complications could be added here. The complications on this list would be more generic,

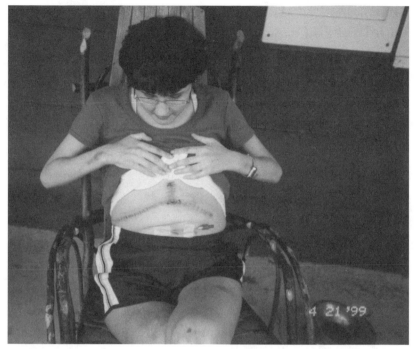

Jessica Hawk-Manus displays her liver transplant scar one and a half months after her March 1999 operation. Her g-tube, visible just above the waistband of her shorts, would remain in place for another six months.

more commonplace to the general population, yet often assaulting those who have CF at an earlier age than one might otherwise expect: gastroesophageal reflux disease (GERD), hypoglycemia, gastroparesis, asthma, and allergies. If you were to ask a person with CF what else they have, the list could be long.

NOTES

1. Lucille Packard Children's Hospital at Stanford, "Respiratory Disorders—Cystic Fibrosis and the Respiratory System: How does cystic fibrosis (CF) affect the respiratory system," www.lpch.org/diseaseHealthInfo/HealthLibrary/respire/cfrespir.html.

2. Medfacts, "Cystic Fibrosis and *Burkholderia Cepacia (B. Cepacia)*," www.njc.org/medfacts/cystic.html.

3. Antoinette Moran, "Cystic Fibrosis-related Diabetes," *CF-Related Diabetes* (October 1996), www.cfservicepharmacy.com/homeline_newsletter/archive.index.cfm?articleid=54.

4. DiabetoValens.com, "Diabetes Matters: Cystic Fibrosis Related Diabetes Mellitus," www.mydiabetovalens.com/infocus/cystic.asp.

5. Moran, "Cystic Fibrosis-related Diabetes."

6. Nishan Wijenaike, Consultant Diabetologist, West Suffolk Diabetes Service, November 2003, www.diabetessuffolk.com.

7. Miles Denton, "MRSA in Cystic Fibrosis [online]," Leeds University Teaching Hospitals, Leeds, UK, May 2001, www.cysticfibrosismedicine.com/htmldocs/CFText/mrsa.htm.

8. Denton, "MRSA in Cystic Fibrosis."

9. ADC Online, "Archives of Diseases in Childhood," adc.bmjjournals.com/cgi/content/abstract/archdischild%3B84/2/160.

10. ADC Online, "Archives of Diseases in Childhood."

11. Norma Kennedy Plourde's Cystic Fibrosis website, personal.nbnet.nb.ca/nnormap/CF.htm or www3.nbnet.nb.ca/normap/cfhistory.htm.

12. Children's Liver Disease Foundation, www.childliverdisease.org/diseases/cyctic.

A Second Chance:
The Lung Transplant

8

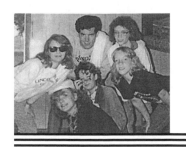

Twenty years have passed since I first went to CF camp. In the mid-1990s, while the disease itself remained incurable, treatments were changing. Perhaps the most seemingly miraculous new option was the double lung transplant. It had worked so well for Mike Maggio, award-winning director of Chicago's Goodman Theater. Maybe it would save some of my friends. I got word in 1993 that my friend Amy Thom had undergone a double lung transplant. I had not realized she had been that sick, so I was surprised. Truly interested in hearing her story, I began to ask Amy about her experiences through a series of letters. "There's a really amazing story here," I thought, "and I want to write about it." So I set out with a tape recorder, notepad, and camera and interviewed Amy and her mother Margaret in what would be the first in a long series of interviews with children and young adults who have CF and their family members. It was also, unbeknownst to me at the time, the beginning of a career for me. Once again CF brought me something special, something that would change my life. Listening to Amy's story I knew I was listening to the tale of a true miracle.

AMY'S MIRACLE

On November 23, 1993, 16-year-old Amy Thom underwent ten hours of lifesaving surgery. Amy's lungs, damaged by cystic fibrosis, were removed and replaced with healthy donor lungs. Time and again a series of post-surgical complications nearly killed Amy. But miracle after miracle, Amy survived. Two years later, when Amy was 18 years old, she and her mother looked back at the ordeal with a realistic and almost easygoing attitude. Amy and her mother both speak of Amy's transplant and the year that followed. Their story of hope and optimism comes to life on the page. After you have read their story you will understand.

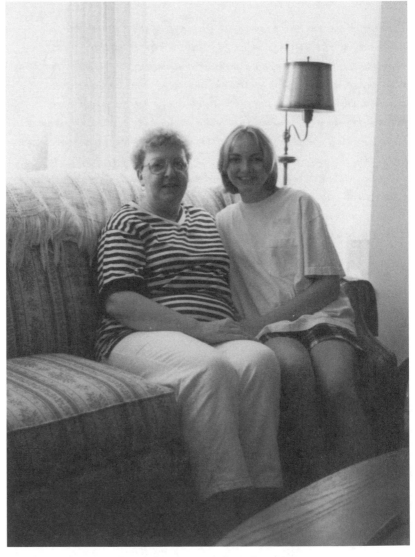

Amy Thom and her mom, Margaret, during the 1995 interview.

AMY: I wasn't too sick until high school. I'd had a port-o-cath to gain weight since seventh grade. So I was still pretty healthy then; I just wasn't gaining weight. I just got progressively worse until I was in the hospital maybe three times a year and then four times a year. By then I wasn't even going to school a full day. I'd come home and sleep, and I'd get up and eat dinner, do my homework, take a bath, and then go back to sleep. I'd get up again in the morning and do my therapy and go to school and come home and sleep all over again. That's all I did. If I wanted to go out, I had to sleep first, or else I'd be too tired. I couldn't do anything. And I was just dying even walking up the stairs at school.

I didn't want to wait until I was so sick that it would have been more risky to have the transplant. I didn't want to get that sick. I didn't want to get to the point like my friend Dawn, who was in bed, who couldn't even walk anymore and was in the hospital like three hundred days out of the year. I didn't want to do that. At first I was struggling with the decision a bit, but then it was just kind of a matter of choosing living over suffocating. I was just going to do it and do it now, and if it doesn't work, oh well! And if it does, cool! I didn't want to get so bad that either it wasn't going to help me or I was just so unhappy that it didn't really matter. I was getting very sick, but I wasn't as sick as a lot of people get. I was getting up there; I could have made it probably a few more years, but I would have been just making it, totally oxygen dependent.

MARGARET: Just before Amy's transplant the doctor said, "I want Amy on oxygen all the time." She was going to have to carry an oxygen tank to school, which she would not do. But she was on oxygen whenever she was home. She had that for about three years. She looked very well; actually, she was deceivingly healthy looking. But when you look at her now comparatively, it's amazing. A lot of people said that Amy always looked transparent, as if her skin had a slight blue tinge to it, not unlike that of skim milk.

AMY: I never thought I looked blue, but I guess I was so used to it that I didn't notice.

141

MARGARET: Amy's sister Katie, who lives on her own, always said, "Mom, she's blue, she's blue." But I didn't notice because I look at her all the time. Katie commented on the color change right away, too. Right after the new lungs were in. "Amy's not blue anymore!"

But as far as thinking about a lung transplant, actually when she was about six years old, they were doing them experimentally in Canada. Amy was always reading and hearing about things about CF. She told her doctor then, "I want one of those." They were doing heart-lung transplants then. "I want that," she said, "I think that's a good idea."

AMY: I was thinking, well can't they just do lungs? Back then it just seemed really simple, like, just give me new lungs!

MARGARET: She thought that was a neat idea, but at the time, of course, we never realized that in fact it would happen.

AMY: It was just too late for me to use DNAse because I had so much scarring in my lungs that it would not have helped. Because of the extent of the damage to the vessels in my lungs, the DNAse might have caused more bleeding because it thins the mucus so much. It works for a lot of people who don't really cough up blood. The therapy vest would have been too harsh; I would have coughed up blood from that, too. I was just kind of stuck.

MARGARET: She was hooked up to nighttime IV feedings for four and a half years prior to the transplant. The port-o-cath is almost like an IV, but it's in the big vessel, so it doesn't come out like an IV. They gave her lipids, hyperal (hyperal is like an amino acid solution), sugars, and a high percentage of glucose, so there are a lot of calories going into the body. If you tried to put all that through a vein in the arm it would be too damaging. All the fluids and high concentration of calories and fatty solutions and calories are absorbed directly into the blood stream. With the port-o-cath she could also get antibiotics at home and IVs at the hospital. Blood can be drawn from the port-o-cath, too.

AMY: It worked well for me. I'm five feet three and I was probably seventy-five pounds when I started; then I got the tube and I got up to 110 pounds. Now I'm around 108 pounds. I eat a lot.

MARGARET: It is a lot different. She actually likes to eat now. When you have constant infection in the body, food just does not even taste that good.

AMY: You're always swallowing mucus, so you have a lot of mucus in your stomach. That's just what you do when you cough. Kind of like a reflex from when you were little. You don't even notice you are doing it. The mucus just comes up when you cough and then gets swallowed right back down.

There were three days of testing to evaluate me for the transplant. I did a six-minute walk where they measured heart rate and oxygen consumption while I was walking. And, oh God, tons of blood. I don't even know what they tested for. Pulmonary scans. Chest measurements. I got shots that I needed updated. Scans, a total-body scan to check for any kind of infection anywhere. Pulmonary Function tests. An ENT doctor scoped my sinuses. Not everybody does the whole big thing. I don't think my friend Mikey did the whole thing I did. See, some people aren't well enough; some of those tests are really hard. Sometimes there just isn't time. We were back and forth quite a bit that summer for various things. They even checked my vagus nerve. They hooked me up to that monitor, and they had an electrode on my chest that caused me to hiccup. I couldn't complete that test because of my port. They had to use that area and they couldn't, so they just did one side. Apparently, when they take out the old lungs, there's a chance that they could nick the vagus nerve or damage it in some way, so they want to make sure that it's strong before they start. That way if they do damage it, they will know how much damage was done. It was all on computerized graphs. There were lots of things that they did.

MARGARET: Amy didn't have much lung capacity left.

AMY: They also did a test where they measured how many calories I used just breathing. I used two thousand calories a day just lying there breathing. That's why people with cystic fibrosis can't gain weight. I needed five to six thousand calories a day just to gain weight. That's why I was on the IV feedings at home because you can't consume that many calories just by eating. You just can't!

MARGARET: She would just move the food around on the plate and her dad would get so upset because we wanted her to eat. You always feel like if they eat they're doing better. Now her friends even comment when they go out. Amy will even say, "Let's go for tacos," and they just look at her and say, "We can't believe that you're eating like this." She was never interested in food before.

AMY: I'm gaining weight gradually.

MARGARET: She was eighty pounds when she came home from the lung transplant. Now she's up to almost 110 and that's without being on any supplements or IVs. A lot of that is muscle weight, which is good. She works out to keep her muscles toned up.

AMY: So I got a transplant. I waited on the list for about three months. I waited until August, after camp, to get on the list. I didn't have a call where they send you back home. Sometimes they will call you to come to the hospital, but at the last minute, they will decide the lungs aren't good enough, so they send you back home.

Most people are in the hospital when they get called for their new lungs. I don't know why that is—probably because we spend so much time in the hospital. I wasn't in Loyola yet; I was still in Wylers. I got called around eleven o'clock at night. Mom was at work and I called my dad and said, "You have to call Mom because . . . and I'll meet you at Loyola." He was just like, "Oh, ok." I called my friend Mikey. His mom answered and I said, "Is Mike there?" and she's like, "Oh, well he's sleeping." I said, "Oh, well I'm leaving for Loyola." She said,

"Just a minute, I'll go get him." He got on the phone and he was like, "Wha—? Ok, go, alright." It was funny.

MARGARET: She went in around one or two o'clock in the morning. They gave her a breathing treatment, and she got some antirejection drugs before she went in. Generally they go back in and open the chest again at least two or three times after the initial surgery because of bleeding. [Note: Since Amy's transplant, this is no longer common practice, although each transplant case is different.] The bleeding is from the vessel that hasn't been clamped off. When they take out cystic lungs, they are very sclerosed and very adhered to the chest wall. As the surgeon put it, they almost have to chisel them out. I asked the surgeon what her lungs looked like. He said, "Like any end-stage cystic lungs look like." When he said "end-stage," I knew that she had not had that much longer to live. So I knew we had done the right thing. I asked what end-stage lungs look like and he said very bulbous, over inflated, sclerosed, and hard. There is no elasticity left.

So all the damage they do to the chest wall, trying to get those old lungs out causes a seeping type of bleeding. Like an oozing in the chest wall. That builds up and they have to open the chest again. They flush all the blood out with saline, and then they have a powder that they put in there that tends to help cauterize the area. But sometimes it takes two or three times before all this has subsided. In the meantime the chest pretty much fills up. I remember one time before they took Amy back into surgery, I had gone into the intensive care unit to see her, and then I went back the next hour, and she was blue from the navel up. I was hysterical, like, "Why is she blue?" They said, "Well we're on our way back into surgery with her." They had prepared us for all the things that could happen to her, but you still don't expect any of it to really happen. So transplant recipients generally go through two or three surgeries in the first forty-eight hours or so. They do one lung at a time, so the recipient really would not have to go on a heart-lung machine.

They don't like to put transplant recipients on a heart-lung machine during surgery, but depending on the person's condition or if the operation is lasting too long, sometimes they have to. In Amy's case they had to put her on for a few hours. She was so bloated when she came off that because so much saline was pumped through her, and the blood was coming off into the machine and then it was filtering back into her body. She looked like a balloon when she came back; she didn't look like a person.

The transplant took ten hours. We were asleep some of the time. They took us to a quiet, out-of-the-way lounge where there were couches, and we were lying down part of the time. We were not [really] sleeping; we were just lying there. Just waiting. There was nothing we could do.

AMY: The first thing I remember was my dad, my sister, and my aunt [coming] over to me. I guess that's when they first woke me up or something a few days after the transplant. Then something happened, and they had to put me back under. I basically lost three or four days; all I remember was getting off the machine and starting to get moving. I did everything I swore I would never do in the hospital. I had always been so independent in the hospital, and I did everything normally. So after the transplant I hated not washing my hair. I used to hate seeing people walking around in gowns with no underwear on, all open in the back. Using bedpans—I hated that. But I did it all because I just didn't care. They moved me out of the ICU to a regular floor. It was a transplant floor. Everyone there had had a heart or lung transplant. I was in the hospital for about two and a half weeks. I could not concentrate to watch TV or anything. That lasted for about a month, I guess from all of the anesthesia. You can't focus on anything. You can't focus enough to just lie there and watch TV; you can't read a magazine much less do homework. I couldn't do homework until January. The steroids do that, too. I remember being sore. Mom always had to massage me.

MARGARET: Her back was sore. During her transplant she was in a semi-upright position with her arms up over her head in a halo position tied to a frame for ten hours. So her muscles were killing her. Her back was what she complained about. She never really complained about anything else. That all went well. She had really good initial recovery from the transplant.

AMY: The only hard part was when they took the chest tubes out. That was about a week after the transplant. It didn't hurt exactly, but I thought they would just take things out of me gradually. I woke up from surgery with four IVs. For some reason they weren't even using my port. One IV was a constant blood gas monitor, and there were all these other IVs. Those were just gradually taken out, and so I assumed the tubes would gradually come out too. One day they just said, "We're going to take your chest tubes out." A bunch of them came in and they were pressing on it and they had me breathe and they said, "Ok, take a deep breath in and let it out." And then they just pulled it out in a rip, and I felt like they were ripping my lung out! It was so weird. I was really shocked; I did not expect that at all. I was shaking. They didn't stitch it. They just put staples in, and that's basically what they are because when they take them out, they use a staple remover like you would use in school. It didn't hurt at all; it's just funny. That was easy, so I didn't think anything else would be hard. They did one and then a few days later they did the other.

MARGARET: We went shopping the day we left the hospital. She came home from the hospital and I felt like a wreck. It was Christmastime and she had to stop at TJMaxx. I said, "Please put your mask on," and Amy said, "I am not putting my mask on." I said, "You just got out of the hospital!" We hadn't even hit the house yet and she was shopping!

When Amy came home it was hard. Her muscles were so weak from the steroids that she had a hard time going up and down the stairs. She went up and down once a day. I almost had to carry her if she had to go up again.

AMY: Getting in the bathtub was a challenge. I could get in, but to get out I had to crawl over the top and go over to the toilet and pull myself up. If I was sitting down I could not lift myself up with just my legs. I had to push with my arms. At that time my niece Allison was a baby. One day we were babysitting her, and I had her in my arms. Mom had to go get the phone and Allison was crying; I had to get the bottle, but I couldn't move. I was just stuck there with this baby in my arms. That was hard, the weakness from the steroids.

MARGARET: One morning Amy woke up and she started crying. She said, "I thought I was going to feel so much better right away, and I feel terrible!" That was the only time Amy ever cried. She just felt so tired and weak. Everyone's story is so different. One of the fellahs, a lawyer named David, who had gotten a transplant before Amy, felt great. He got up from his transplant, and a couple days later he was eating a fried chicken dinner in the hospital, but Amy couldn't even eat at all. Then he left the hospital and stopped for pie and coffee and went home and never had an ounce of problem. Amy was so weak they put an NG (nasogastric) tube down her nose to feed her a liquid formula. She had to keep a lot of calories in her body for the healing; that was what they were concerned about. But then as she started to feel a little better, she did start to eat.

AMY: I was an emotional wreck. The drugs messed me up for a while. They made me edgy and moody for a while. Not mean, just edgy. But that all passed. They do tell you those things may happen. They don't happen to everybody, but they do happen.

MARGARET: Everything seemed to be going well for Amy. Then she came up with this very, very rare complication, which really sent us off into another direction.

AMY: I remember it was sometime in December. I was sitting in the kitchen doing something, and all of a sudden, I couldn't see out of one eye. It was all blurry, and out of one eye was this kaleidoscope vision. This had happened to me before when I had been on birth control pills for regulating my period. I would get this really weird kaleidoscope vision, and then I would get this awful headache. It was just from the hormones, and I had to quit taking the pill. So that's what I thought maybe it was, except that I was not on the pill anymore. I called my dad in and said, "Dad, look at my eye. Is anything wrong with it?" He said, "No, it's fine." Then the sensation just went away. I never got the headache or anything. School was starting at the beginning of January. I was ready, and I wanted to try going back. I went to bed the Sunday night before school started Monday. But I didn't wake up. Or rather I don't remember waking up for another couple of days.

MARGARET: We heard this funny noise in the morning. I thought it was the mourning doves outside. They have this strange, shrill coo. Jerry (Amy's dad) said, "Gee, the mourning doves sound funny this morning." We were lying there and then I said, "I think it's Amy." Jerry said, "What would Amy be doing?" We ran upstairs, and there she was having a seizure. She was still in bed, and by the time I got up there she was totally flaccid; she didn't move. She was comatose; she didn't respond in any way at all. I thought she'd had a stroke because, on rare occasions, it has been recorded that the immunosuppressants can cause a stroke. Or it can cause a person to seize from them anyway. I just panicked. I didn't know what to think. She wasn't responding to me. We dialed 911 and the ambulance came. Actually, we would have been better off to take her to the hospital ourselves because we spent forty-five minutes in the ambulance while they tried to get an IV line started on her. She had very bad veins at that point from so many years of IVs. I kept saying, "Let's just go! She's got a central line. We'll get it started when we get into the emergency room." I'm a nurse, so I know a little about what to do. I kept telling the ambulance drivers, "Please let's go, or I'm going to take her myself." They would not pay any attention to me. She had a couple more seizures in the ambulance, but finally we got there. By that time she was responding, but she was totally off the wall. We could not make any sense of what she was saying. She didn't know anything that was going on. She had another seizure in the ER.

We briefed the ER staff on what had been going on with Amy. They had no idea. We told them we had to get her to Loyola right away. They did a CAT scan while we were there. The CAT scan was negative. They said her brain was fine and nothing was wrong. Well that was wrong. We got to Loyola and they got her under control after she had some more seizures there. She had an MRI and that showed that she had these lesions in her brain.

A few days went by, and she was controlled on antiseizure medicine. She came out of it, and she was fine. The first few days she was a bit wild, but that was just a reaction from the seizures. She went through a bunch of tests, but no one knew what the lesions were. They look like this, they said, or they look like that. Everyone had their own theory of what they were, and finally they concluded that it was toxoplasmosis. There was one titer that came back weakly positive for that, so that's what they concluded it was. They put her on high doses of sulfa drugs and a couple other pills.

That went on for two months. She was doing fine, but she didn't return to school. She had a tutor come to the house. They kept checking the lesions on the MRI. They did not get bigger, but they got denser. They kept saying they had to go into her brain and do surgery. Amy's dad was really, really worried about that. He thought they were going to slip or something.

AMY: I was just like, do it! Go in there. I was tired of it.

MARGARET: She also had a couple of periods of mild rejection, and she went back for a bronchoscopy. With rejection you get this kind of cough that you don't even really notice. They just know if it's rejection from the biopsy. They go down your throat and take some bits of tissue from the lung and then they know.

AMY: I didn't feel sick. I did feel a little bit more tired, and I'd get a bit of a hacky cough that progressively got worse. For a while I got checked for that once a month. I'd had a few small episodes where I was on three-day IV steroids at home. Then I had a really big episode of rejection when I was getting the biopsy, where they had to put a catheter in the vein in my groin and take plasmapheresis. That's where they take the plasma off your blood supply. It's like dialysis. They filter the plasma, and they put some kind of protein on it to trick the immune system into thinking it's not going to reject it. It worked.

MARGARET: At one point late in February they noticed a bit of rejection, and they put her back in the ICU. That time they decided to go in and do what they call a closed brain biopsy, where they just drill a burr hole, and they go in and draw a sample of the lesion.

AMY: I was awake for that. I remember that that was real scary. They were giving me anesthesia, and they started shaving my head and telling me I was going to feel that my head was numb up here. Then before they started drilling I'm like, "I'm still awake!" but they just brushed it off and started drilling my head! I remember this! The doctor was drilling through my skull. I started crying because I was kind of out of it since I had been drugged. I was really nervous, but I remember it, and the surgeon said, "Amy you're going to have to stop crying." I said, "I'm still awake!" He told the anesthesiologist, "Give her some more!" The anesthesiologist said, "I've already given her more than . . . ." The surgeon said, "I don't care. Give it to her."

MARGARET: They got a sample of the lesion out, but they did not get enough to make an accurate diagnosis. So they still did not know what was going on. Amy came home and a couple more weeks went by. She had to go back into the hospital for some more rejection problems. Then we made the decision. They said, "It's got to be done; she's got to have a craniotomy. We've got to go in there and see what these are because they're growing." So they went in, and they did a craniotomy. They shaved the whole right side of her head and did two openings, one on the top of the skull and one in the back.

AMY: He asked me if I wanted them to shave my whole head because they had to shave a lot. I asked them to leave some hair, so that if I put a hat on, it would look like I had some hair. He said, "Alright, alright, alright." So he parted it and shaved it. Later, I would just throw a hat on and pull my hair through the back, and I looked like I had hair.

MARGARET: She was adorable.

AMY: Then they did the craniotomy. I remember I talked the minute I came out of it. Before surgery they thought I was either going to end up with weakness on one side or my speech would be messed up. But I was fine. I remember one of the nurses and the doctors were saying something about me, and I knew the answer, so I answered them. I don't think they really listened to me.

MARGARET: They took out two lesions. That's all there were. They discovered these lesions were a fungus called aspergillosis that a lot of us have in our airways and in our sinuses. That is where Amy's probably came from. But when you're on immunosuppressants, you never know what the body might react to. So she was on immunosuppressants, and her immune system shut way down. This particular little fungus got into her blood stream and traveled. Usually it stays systemic, and they treat you for it if they find it in your blood. But hers traveled to her brain and made these little lesions that encapsulated themselves. This is very, very rare. Usually this spreads. They said that out of maybe twenty-one people reported as having this in their brain only seven have lived, and that's only because they caught it in the first week and they found it, because it spreads. But somehow Amy encapsulated it, so they turned into lesions, and it didn't spread. All the infection stayed in this small area. They were able to get them out intact. We've heard in passing being told to med students, "this is the girl." Apparently she's the only person on record who survived these for two months, untreated.

AMY: Then I went on an antifungal medicine called Amphotericin which is supposed to be really bad. They call it amphoterrible because people have really bad reactions to it. We were warned about kidney failure and liver failure.

MARGARET: The infectious disease doctor painted a very bleak picture for my husband and me. He said, "She must go on this because it has to save her life." She had to be on this Amphotericin-B IV every day for three months. It is very potent, so they have to give it in divided doses. The doctor said that it would definitely cause kidney damage and that she might even end up getting dialysis. So we're like, oh my God what next? This kid is just . . . it just went from one thing to another.

But again she defied all of their predictions. She never had any problems. None at all. But through this Amy didn't know that her odds were not good at all. She knew there was a problem because we had to draw blood from her port two or three times a day and take it into the hospital. They would do the testing and fax the info back to Loyola. They checked her kidney functions very closely; two times a week it was checked. They were right on top of it, but it was a real precarious problem. But she has no kidney damage. All her kidney functions are fine.

AMY: I was an emotional wreck that whole time with the brain and just everything. I was so mad! I had done all this just to live, and here I was getting better and then the brain thing comes out of the blue, and, of course, I'm the only one who has ever had it, so no one knows what it is. Then during all of this, my friend Mikey died, and it was like, what next? Everything! If I had not done the transplant I still would have died. I had wanted the transplant, but that was all we bargained for. They tell you infection is a big risk, but I think we were all thinking in terms of surgical infection. I was never thinking a brain infection. I always thought it would be something to do with my lungs that would be the big problem.

All the episodes with rejection and the brain surgery were between the end of December and the beginning of March. I'm still on antirejection drugs, and I always will be. It's kind of like cancer in remission; the further out you get, the more optimistic they are. I haven't had a biopsy in quite awhile, six months maybe.

I finished my junior year of high school in July 1994 with a tutor because I had dropped a couple of classes. By then my hair was growing out, so before I started school, I was able to get it all cut. It was cut in a short, boyish style at this time last year. I took a summer school class, and they let me wear the baseball cap in school, even though it was against the dress code. It didn't look too bad, kind of like a weird cut, like I did it on purpose. It had been bad at first because I had two big scars and staples and stitches. It just looked awful, so I kept the hat on then.

[My transplant] scar goes side to side under my breasts. Under my arms is pretty much numb and my right breast is numb. I doubt the numbness will go away because it has been a while. I think the nerve damage is permanent. They did not tell me to expect that. But it is not a big deal. It's just numb. It doesn't hurt or anything. I have three scars from the transplant alone. Then two port scars and two brain surgery scars.

MARGARET: She started her senior year and sailed right through it.

AMY: Now I still worry, but I don't think about it as much. When I was in eighth grade, I didn't think that I'd make it to my sixteenth birthday. But then I was 16 and driving a car, so then I thought I would not graduate from high school. I didn't think I would go to college. Before I got my transplant, I always expected to die because people around me died. It's weird now not to expect to die. I still have cystic fibrosis, but it's different now. It's still there, but my lungs don't have it. The one part, the bad part. The new lungs will never get it because it's genetic, and the new lungs don't have that genetic defect; it's someone else's genes really. The only part of CF I have is the pancreatic insufficiency, so I still take Pancrease when I eat. I have CF because I still have sinus problems and the digestive problems. Every now and then I have a little hacky cough from my sinuses, but that's it.

MARGARET: With cystic fibrosis there is always a chance you could become diabetic because all the ducts to the pancreas become blocked. It's highly unlikely that'll happen to Amy now because she hasn't gotten diabetes already. There could be some liver problems. There will always be a few things that she will have to be on the alert for, and she will always have to take her digestive enzymes.

We have a lot more time since Amy had her transplant. Our lives and our whole family's lives have changed considerably. CF involves so many systems of the body, so there is just so much to do to keep them well. Over the years that really becomes the biggest concentration of your life. It just takes over your whole life whether you want it to or not. You try not to let it, but it does. It's the center of everything because this child has so many problems, and you have to deal with them. Yet Amy never complained; it never bothered her all that much. She maintained as much normalcy to her life as she could.

Just so she could get through coughing, which could take forty-five minutes, then throwing up, and breakfast, Amy had to get up at five-thirty in the morning to go to school. There were so many of those things that went on for years and years that were just part of life. We didn't really think about it because what else could she do? It would take her almost two and a half hours to get ready for school in the morning by the time she got her therapy and coughed, threw up, and then tried to eat breakfast even though she didn't want it. The last few years when she had the IV, she had to unhook the IV and flush the port. Everything took time. Most kids can jump up at eight o'clock in the morning, throw their clothes on, have toast, and go. Amy, and any kid who has a lot to do like she did every morning, just takes a lot of time. A lot of people wondered why Amy was having a lung transplant. Because she looked so great, they figured how could she be that sick? That was deceiving because she never really looked that ill. She knew, and we knew. We knew what to look for but others didn't.

AMY: I take thirty pills in the morning. There's Cyclosporine, which is the antirejection, and Sporonox, which is antifungal; Dilantin, the antiseizure drug, which I don't think I need, but they don't want to take me off of that yet; Pancrease; vitamins; steroids every other day; and high blood pressure medicine because of the Cyclosporine. I take about fifteen pills at lunch. It only takes me two swallows. The Dilantin lowers the Cyclosporine, so there is a little bit of a problem keeping the Cyclosporine level high enough. It is all well watched. And I take three puffs a day of inhaled steroids for antirejection, too.

MARGARET: I feel really fortunate and really blessed that we had extremely good doctors. That's a big factor—people who had such great knowledge that we were able to do this. I'm really glad that we had the opportunity to know these people who helped Amy. It just seemed that everything just kept falling into place, and everyone took great care of her.

It's really quite an experience to know that someone else's lungs are in Amy's body, and that they are functioning and that life definitely goes on. When you get into this organ transplant scenario, you really know what life is. It's hard to get lungs. People who have CF are usually small, so they need small lungs. The lungs are going to be from a teenager, or a child, or a very small adult. Children are usually killed in auto accidents, and so there is crushing injury and the lungs can't be used. A lot of the lungs come from children who have committed suicide because there is no damage to the chest. I had a little bit of a hard time with that.

AMY: I don't know what happened to the person whose lungs I got. They said she had a head injury. I think she was a little younger than I am. I wrote the family a letter a while ago before I graduated. I think I started off by saying that in a couple of days I'm going to graduate. I related the whole letter to that. I just have to get it to them. All we have to do is send it to one of our pulmonary nurses, and she'll forward it to them. They're from the Chicagoland area. I don't know anything about them, and I don't know if they know anything about me. If they wanted to know me, that would be fine, and I'd do it, but I don't feel like I've got to know who it is. I do not want to upset the family.

MARGARET: She just wants them to know the good that came out of this for her. It's been quite an experience. Major surgery and brain surgery, which is pretty critical stuff. I have to think that there is a reason all this transpired. We have had so many friends who have not made it and then so many who have. There is no explanation, and I don't know why. I'm glad it turned out the way it did, of course. It's changed our whole lives. I'm still recovering! It happened so fast.

AMY: Now I can swim. I could never swim before. I didn't even know how to swim because I never really could learn since the chlorine would make me cough up blood. I was always nervous being around chlorine, so I never went in the water. Swimming is just more excessive than you think, and I would have gotten too tired. Now I can just jump on in and do whatever I want, and it's weird.

MARGARET: Amazing things happen. Even the clubbing in Amy's fingers subsided—reversed. There's probably a slight clubbing; they're still thick, and they'll never completely reverse. But that was a surprise. The doctors did not expect it, at first. Her CF doctor at the University of Chicago is overwhelmed by it all; she just looks at her, and she'll just say, "Never in my wildest dreams did I think someone could go through this." She's delighted.

AMY: I visit my nurses because I actually miss going into the hospital, and I miss my old nurses. When I visit I don't get to see all of them because some of them are night shift nurses. So I sent them my graduation announcement.

MARGARET: Before the transplant, Amy had really become dependent on me for a lot of things. I had to do a lot for her. At the end there, she could only come down the stairs in the morning and go back up at night. If she forgot something, she could not make it upstairs again, before her lung transplant. She just couldn't do the stairs, and afterward, for a little while, it was the same way.

AMY: Now I just run!

MARGARET: One day she came down and said, "Do you realize I just ran up those stairs Mom? And I'm not even huffing and puffing!" It was so amazing.

AMY: Now I just run . . .

About a year after this interview, Amy began to feel poorly. Assuming she had the flu, Amy pushed on, not wanting to miss out on any of the events in her typically busy life of college, work, and spending time with her friends. When her flu-like symptoms lingered longer than they should have, tests revealed that Amy's body was rejecting her new lungs. As her new lungs became stiffer, it became increasingly more difficult for Amy to breathe and to function normally. Unwilling to give up, Amy decided to try for a second double lung transplant and was re-listed. Amy agreed to a tracheotomy and was placed on a ventilator, which would help her damaged lungs breathe while she awaited another transplant. Amy was admitted to a ventilator care facility where she remained on the ventilator. Amy died on July 25, 1997, two and a half weeks after her 20th birthday, roughly a year after her first rejection symptoms appeared.

NEW LUNGS FOR MELISSA: A LIVING DONOR

Melissa Kay Reta celebrated her 30th birthday on May 7, 2004. Born with meconium ileus, she was diagnosed with CF at five days old. Her family considers the early diagnosis a lucky thing because they were able to treat her from the beginning, which they feel helped her to stay as healthy as she was for so long. After Melissa's birth and diagnosis, she was not hospitalized again until she was 19½ years old, when she was admitted for her first case of pneumonia and her first round (of many) of IV therapy. She did not colonize *pseudomonas* until she was 21. That was what caused her health to start to decline, says her mother. In February 2000, Melissa was in the process of being evaluated for transplant and was found to be culturing aspergillosis. Thus her rapid decline and need for transplant had begun. Early in April 2000, Melissa met with a team of doctors that told her she was a viable candidate for transplant. At the same meeting they discussed the possibility of a living donor transplant. Melissa spent her 26th birthday in the hospital waiting for her transplant. She was unable to blow out even two candles on her cake. On May 24, 2000, Melissa received her living donor transplant. One lobe was donated by her uncle, and the other came from a male friend of her family. Her surgery began at 7:00 a.m. and was over by 10:30 a.m. Since Melissa had a living donor transplant, three people were in surgery at the same time.

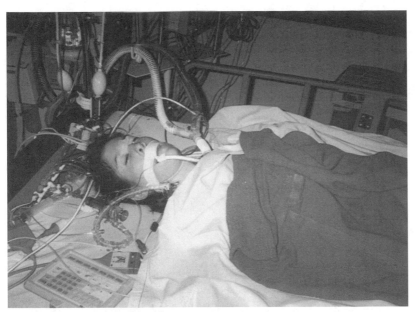

One of the first photos taken of Melissa Kay Reta when her family was allowed to see her after surgery.

After surgery, Melissa was in the Intensive Care Unit (ICU) for five days. Her family had been told she would sleep through the night, but she woke up at 11:00 p.m. the same night of her surgery. A small portable fan was placed on Melissa's bed, and her feet were covered with cold rags because the medications she was on caused her body to feel very hot. Melissa remembers that while she was on the ventilator, she felt as if she were on the edge of losing control. The endotracheal tube in her throat (which connected her to the ventilator) made her feel like she was constantly gagging.

The ventilator and the drainage tubes from her chest were the worst things Melissa had to deal with during the entire episode. A couple days after the transplant Melissa was wheeled into the hallway for her first walk. It took twenty minutes to load all of her equipment onto the IV pole just for her five-minute walk. Just four days after surgery, and still in the ICU, Melissa told her mother, "Mom, I need a bucket, a razor, and some shaving cream. Just because one has a transplant does not mean one has to have hairy legs!"

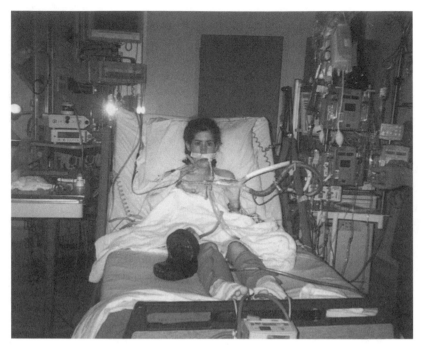

Melissa awake and still on the ventilator.

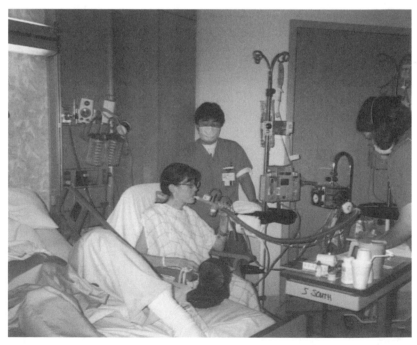

Out of the ICU, Melissa takes one of the many respiratory therapy treatments she received every day.

She was released to go home twenty-one days after her surgery. Her doctors told her she was a textbook example of how they would like all lung transplant surgery recoveries to go. When you have a lobar transplant like Melissa did—that is the transplant of one lobe of each lung rather than two entire lungs—the new lungs are so much smaller than the previous lungs that, immediately following surgery, the rib cage begins to shrink to surround the new lungs for protection. At the same time the new lungs are expanding to fill up the rib cage space. This is a natural process, but it surprised doctors when lobar transplants were first being done. Melissa's family saw the first set of X-rays three days after her surgery, and they could not tell that she had only two lobes instead of a full set of lungs (five lobes)! Everyone was amazed, says Melissa's mother, by how quickly the lobes expanded and the rib cage shrank to meet them.

On the one hundredth day after Melissa's transplant, her family made her a cake with one hundred candles ablaze on top. She blew out every single one! Today, almost four years after surgery, the transplant team at University of Southern California's University Hospital in Los Angeles is comprised of the leading surgeons worldwide with the best statistics for living lobar transplants. The surgeon and his team give seminars, speeches, and conferences locally and worldwide to teach others about this type of transplant and surgery. They use Melissa's X-rays to tell the story.

Did this transplant change Melissa's life? "You bet it did!" says her mother. Now she can sing and laugh, be independent again, walk without coughing, dance and kiss her husband without coughing, dream about her future . . . and she can breathe!

Since surgery, Melissa has met with many medical dilemmas, but she is very proactive with her health, never missing a beat when she thinks something is wrong. Although she has come up against some very difficult and unusual side effects from surgery, they have all been remedied, and once she is good to go again, she is off and running! Since her transplant, Melissa has been busy cramming as much living into her life and as much life into her living as possible! She has driven a race car at a speed of 176 miles per hour; she's traveled around the United States for vacations and lung transplant conferences and even to Hawaii to serve as maid of honor in her best friend's wedding. She walks the walk-a-thons; volunteers to speak about lung transplants and organ donations; served as a board member on Second Wing, a lung transplant organization, for a year; and co-organized a conference the organization held in San Diego in 2002. She ran a relay race at the 2002 Transplant Olympics in Florida and was honored when the Olympic organization asked her to speak to an audience of over five hundred living donors, recipients, and family members. The transplant team at USC calls Melissa to come talk to newly admitted patients and their families who are there to have transplants. There is nothing Melissa would not do for an interested person who she feels has something to learn from her experience—including lifting her shirt and showing her scar, which she wears proudly! She has made so many new and wonderful friends because of this experience. There was a time in Melissa's life when she thought her life was over. Now that she has been given a second chance, she does not let any opportunity to experience life to the fullest pass her by.

Did You Know?
Writer, producer, and famous *Psycho* director, Alfred Hitchcock (1899–1980), known as the master of suspense, had a granddaughter who has had a lung transplant because she has CF.[1]

WAITING . . . AND WAITING . . . AND WAITING

While the transplant and the following recovery might seem tough to endure, sometimes just waiting for a lung transplant can be a harrowing experience:

"Can you believe this? Today, my twentieth day on the transplant list, I got my second call telling me a donor had been found. My first call came on December 29 after only ten days of waiting. Those lungs turned out not to be suitable for transplant. Well, this morning, when the transplant coordinator called to tell me that they had another donor, I told her about the sore throat I had. She told me that she was going to call the surgeon and call me back. After a few minutes, she called and told me that since I didn't have a fever and felt fine otherwise, the surgeon didn't think there would be a problem. I was told to come to the hospital quickly, and the transplant team would assess me more closely when I got there.

"Well, I got there, had a few tests, and saw a few doctors. The CF specialist didn't foresee a problem, but the infectious disease specialist said he had serious reservations. He asked me, 'How bad do you need these lungs?' I told him that if the team had any reservations, I would wait. He said he wanted to huddle with the CF specialist and surgeon to discuss things. Eventually, a doctor came in and told me that the team decided not to take a chance because if it turned out that I had a virus, it could be a big risk. After I saw the concern on his face, I was comfortable with that decision. How can I be confident going into surgery if the transplant team isn't? We're going to monitor things over the weekend, and if my chest gets infected, I'll probably have to be admitted to clear it up. At this point, I think I would prefer that."—Gil Stoddard, 29, Toronto

Gil finally received his transplant on February 1, 2004, and now says, "I feel *great!*"

Nineteenth century composer Frederick Chopin could have suffered from cystic fibrosis. Chopin almost defines the idea of the Romantic artist—frail, compassionate, talented, and tragically young at death. Tuberculosis (TB) is sometimes thought of as the Romantic disease, and it did claim many artists in the early nineteenth century. Chopin might have died from tuberculosis, but there is some evidence that he actually suffered from the then-unknown disease cystic fibrosis. Chopin was ill from childhood, and certain traits of his lung disease sound to modern physicians more like cystic fibrosis than common TB.[2]

TRY AND TRY AGAIN

"I first realized that there was a difference between my friends and me when I was about seven years old. I was old enough then to go to sleepovers, but I couldn't go because my friends' parents didn't know how to give me my therapy." Treated for asthma until she was three years old and her true diagnosis was made, 18-year-old Katie Kocelko has already lived an amazing life.

"By the time I was nine years old my CF was pretty bad. I was listed for a transplant." At 10 years old, Katie appeared to be the picture of health with a radiant tan and sun-streaked blonde hair. Yet, she had much to worry about, much more than the average 10-year-old's worries. In fact, much more than even the typical adult's.

Katie's Problems

It's a bright summer morning in 1995 and 10-year-old Katie Kocelko is just finishing up her morning treatment. Her ThAIRapy Vest is pumping away at 14 Hertz and the aerosol mask on her face is marked with a piece of masking tape on which the word "DNAse" has been written. In Katie's own words, this is cystic fibrosis from the perspective of a 10-year-old who already knows how to tell it like it is.

"Some CF patients don't have a button," Katie begins, referring to her g-tube. "Every once in a while you have to get it changed. And it does kind of hurt when you get it changed. This one is smaller. It seems like it's higher up but it's not. Before it was that big round one that had to be coiled up and taped to my stomach. I got it in October when I was still 9. It hurt the first couple days. But then it turned out to be a real success. I gained a lot of weight. I was gaining about a pound a week. Now as I do the tube feedings, I'm less hungrier in the day, so I don't eat as much as I used to do. I used to throw up all the time, but now I don't because they gave me Cisapride. It helps my stomach settle down so I don't throw it [the food] up. I take it half an hour before I eat or do my feedings. I take enzymes for my feedings. I'm going to start taking them more than once during a feeding because I will get more nutrition that way. I usually wake up to go to the bathroom in the middle of the night, always at the same time, around four o'clock in the morning. So when I wake up I might take more then. So it might be by my bedside. I put the feeding on hold for a second and unhook it when I go to the bathroom. When you have to go to the bathroom, you have to do things quickly. I don't do my tube feedings when I go to sleepovers, unless it's going to be for a while. Like, I took it to St. Louis with me. We were there from Sunday to Friday.

"I had that skin thing," Katie said, again referring to her g-tube. "I don't know what you call it. There was extra skin there and you have to burn it off. I have the package right here: silver nitrate. About three months ago, I wasn't changing my button and they never told me to change it. I asked my Mom, 'Shouldn't I change it now? It's been awhile.' She said, 'Well you're not gaining enough weight.' I said, 'I thought you had to change it every once in a while whether you gain weight or not.' You're supposed to because all the enzymes eat the rubber away, and it makes a hole in there. And there was a hole, and one night it was hooked on something, and I sat up and it pulled out. I put my hand on it, and I felt there was nothing there. It didn't hurt because the balloon was busted. My mom got a new one, and that one had a teeny hole that she couldn't see, so it fell out again when I was lifting my brother's bag. It was so heavy; I just heaved the bag up and my button went flying with it. My mom wasn't home, so I did it alone. The skin kind of globbed in, so it looked like it was already healed, but it wasn't. You couldn't see anything in there because the skin kind of pushed in, and it looked like it was already starting to close up. But I didn't look at it the other time; I just covered it up.

"I don't wear bikinis because it hurts and also because you can see it. I have kind of tight bathing suits, so you can see the bump. If people ask what it is, I just tell them I had an operation. That's not really lying. I'm just not telling the whole thing. It doesn't hurt when I swim. Some people go on water slides and they go on their belly, and I can't do that. I was on my slip and slide and I fell on my stomach and it started to bleed. I cleaned it up and it was ok. It only bleeds where that extra skin is.

"I used to take tumbling. I could still, if I wanted to, but I couldn't at first. I still do gymnastics at home. I still play around. The thing that I don't like is I can't do [as much] as other kids. I can't go outside and run around because I cough a lot. The weather's too hot. I can't have as many sleepovers. I can't have as much fun. I go outside swimming a lot, but there's not a lot to do outside. This is a particularly bad summer. Last year was cooler; it wasn't really hot till August.

"I get in trouble a lot for not doing my treatments. I do the Vest. Sometimes when it's really busy, I do it in the morning and at night. But now I do it three times a day. In the morning I do one when I get up at nine or ten o'clock, and I do my Albutrol neb and my DNAse neb, and I do my Tobra. I take Cipro twice a day in the morning and at night. It's that big round pill that says 250 on it. That's an antibiotic. And then I like my Flintstones vitamins. They taste really good. I like the orange the best. I use two liters of oxygen when I sleep, but sometimes it's a little more or less because my little brother likes to play around with the machine. I just use it when I need it. I've been using it more right now. The oxygen machine makes too much noise and keeps me awake, so it's downstairs in the living room. The tubing goes all the way down there from my room. I'm going back into the hospital this week because I'm doing worse. My mom says I should just go in now and get it over with before my baby brother's christening.

"Usually I just say I have asthma. Then, later on if I can trust them, I can tell them I have CF. I do have asthma, but it comes and goes with wheezing and stuff. They don't get mad at me because I lied because I just didn't tell them everything. There's this one girl and she's a big tattletale; she tells everybody. It was ok. Everyone in the fourth grade knows. My teacher knows. She'll eventually tell them if I don't tell them. The first time I go in the hospital she'll probably tell them. They'll ask why I was gone so long. Then when I come back, everyone tells me why I go in the hospital. They know I have CF; I just tell them I have to go in every once in a while because I get sick. I have one best friend who I can really trust. We've been friends for three years. I usually tell her everything. I tell her if I get really sick. I told her when I went in to get my button. I tell her that I get new ones and how they have to change it. She's seen it. She thinks it's cool to have a friend with CF.

"I don't have any friends who have CF. Nobody in my school that I know of has CF. Some kids have asthma but none of them have CF.

"I can look into the future. I'm going to walk on the moon! No, I'm not. I'm just kidding. I'm going to live till I'm 100. I'm going to be a doctor maybe; I'm not sure yet. I want to work at a hospital. Or maybe I'll be a model. I want to get married and have maybe two kids, all girls—five girls! I'm going to go to college.

"St. Louis was good; I went with Mom and Dad and the little baby, Michael. He was still on breast milk. My little brother John went to my Grandma's, and my older brother Stephan went to our cousins' house. I thought I was just going to be in the hospital because they told me I'd have to stay there. It was for three days. It was different there. They had TVs that weren't on the wall; they were right next to you, and you could move them around like right in front of you. I was on the seventh floor, the surgical floor for lung transplants. The nurses there were very nice. You shared one phone with your roommate. It wasn't like our phones [at Children's Memorial Hospital]; it was a regular normal phone.

"Some of the tests were ok. Some of them were hard. I'd have to say my worst test was when they had to put some dye in me. They gave me a shot up here [on my arm] where they give you blood tests; it was like an IV, and it had to stay in there for just a little bit to put the dye in. It stinged a lot. It was sore. But that was the hardest part. Then all I had to do was sit there. They were looking at my lungs and how many scars and stuff. There was a screen, and all the white stuff was scars and the black stuff was my lungs. I would see it, but I had to lie down most of the time. I got to watch *The Land before Time*, too. It was a long test. They measured my height and my chest size. At the end Dr. Mallory told me about some stuff. That to get the lung transplant you had to be the same height and the same blood type. He told me I was an A blood type. He said if I got really bad, my parents, if they had the same blood type, could give me a lower lobe [each donating from one of their lungs]. That was just an idea. I had a lot of blood tests. Well, I had one where there were at least ten tubes they had to fill up. I had to ride a bike and all these wires were connected to me. I had this thing around my forehead, and I had to breathe through a mask. I just had to breathe regular air through the mask. They were just measuring how I was breathing. I didn't like the mask because I couldn't breathe really easy with that. I did good when I was biking. I would have done better if I didn't have the mask. I did PFTs. Their machine was different. Ours shows the breath going in a circle; theirs shows a line just straight across. I didn't really care about the tests. I just did the best I could on everything. I got a lot of prizes from everybody. I got a lot of stickers. I got a collection of stickers for three days. I got two and a half pages full of stickers. They're those hospital stickers that Children's used to have. We went to Great America and the big Science Center. I have to go to the hospital in St. Louis every six months, so I'll be back in December just for a regular checkup. We're going to go back to the Science Center because we didn't get to finish it.

"They said I need a lung transplant and they're going to put me on the list. They said I was fifth or sixth in my height and blood type. They said sometime next year maybe. They said try to keep yourself as healthy as possible and do your treatments right, and they put me on an exercise program. I haven't started yet because I don't know where the papers are. My mom put them somewhere. I'm supposed to work out my legs and my arms.

"When I go there, we're going to have to live in an apartment while we wait. My mom said we could get a cat as a pet, but Dr. McColley said we can't get a cat. It's kind of hard for me because I'm supposed to go, but my best friend is moving soon. So I think that I'm going to go to St. Louis, and by the time that I come back, she is going to already be moved. She's moving to Colorado.

"They said after the transplant I'd have tubes connected to my lungs to get out all the extra blood. So I might see blood coming out of me. I'm supposed to have a central line. They said I have a choice if I want to keep it in for a while or if I want them to take it out and then put it back in. I'm supposed to keep it when I go home. But they said if I want they could take it out, but they'll have to put it back in.

"They told me that usually everyone lives through the transplant, but dealing with rejection, that's the hardest. Most of the kids they do live. Not very many die. I'm not really sad or, you know, thinking this is my last year of living or something. I think I can do it because I've done a lot of stuff in my life, and this is going to be a big one, but I think I can do it.

"That's really the problems I have. Dealing with friends, the lung transplant, and my button."

Just a year later, Katie was pale, thin, and wearing a nasal cannula for supplemental oxygen. "Right after my eleventh birthday I got new lungs. I thought I'd gotten a miracle cure." In fact, at 11, Katie believed she no longer had CF and would refer to herself in the past saying, "when I used to have CF . . ."

Not a Cure

While the newly transplanted lungs do not and never will have CF, a transplant should not be mistaken for a cure. "It's trading one set of problems for another," said Margaret Thom, Amy's mother. She explained that Amy still had to take a large quantity of pills to ward off rejection, counteract different medicines, and keep her healthy. In addition, she said that she and Amy had

Check with your local CF Foundation chapter for annual fundraising opportunities such as Chicago's Great Strides Walk-a-Thon and the Bowl for Breath Bowl-a-Thon.

known what to expect with CF, but they had not known what to expect in terms of Amy's health and the possible downfalls she might experience with the transplant. This was new territory for Amy and Margaret. When Amy died, her mother felt they had been literally sideswiped.

Katie's Transplant, Take One

Despite the fact that she had been on full-time oxygen for quite some time, "I didn't realize how close I had been to dying," says Katie today. "There's a line between faith and hope and also feeling invincible, like, that can't happen to *me*. But so far I've beat the odds. I've been lucky. My first transplant lasted seven years. I was able to play badminton and do gymnastics, and I finished high school. I would have missed out on seven years of my life if I hadn't gone ahead with the transplant. When I had the transplant, my doctors told me I had a 50 percent chance of surviving five years."

Katie's Transplant, Take Two

Three years post transplant Katie was diagnosed with bronchiolitis obliterans. "My new lungs were being destroyed. So I re-listed for another transplant. The lung damage plateaued at one point and then it dropped, so my status on the transplant list was changed to active." After two years of being back on nebulizer treatments and doing PEP therapy, in the spring of 2003 Katie underwent her second double lung transplant. "My mom and I had to move to St. Louis again while my dad stayed home with my three brothers. The first transplant was only partly covered by insurance," Katie explains, "but my Girl Scout troop and the school PTA helped raise the rest. This time my parents' insurance paid for the whole thing—$350,000. But we had to pay for our apartment in St. Louis and our living expenses. The hospital has special deals with the apartments to get a short-term rate for transplant patients. People who don't have money for this can stay at the Ronald McDonald house. I had to stay in St. Louis for three months after each transplant. Oh, except this time I got to come home for one weekend! I had to go to my senior prom because I was nominated for prom queen!"

"Younger kids don't get second transplants because they don't do well, so I've been told." In order to stay as healthy as possible while she waited for her second transplant, Katie worked to keep her weight up, and she went to physical therapy three times a week. "If I couldn't have had the second transplant, I don't know where I'd be now. I was on oxygen again because I was in chronic rejection, and things were getting worse and worse. I was homeschooled with tutors my senior year of high school. When I went to St. Louis for the transplant, it was up to me to finish my schoolwork on my own, which I did. I really wanted to get the transplant over with so I could go away to college in the fall."

Katie is thriving at Bradley University in Peoria, Illinois, now in the middle of her freshman year. But despite two transplants, her future remains uncertain.

Katie's Transplant, Take Three?

"I'm scared now because I have been told that a second transplant rarely lasts as long as the first. And I've never heard of anyone getting a third transplant. So I wonder if that means that I have less than seven years to live."

Despite her worry, Katie lives life to the fullest. "I am a public relations major. I am mostly taking general education classes right now and a few communication classes. I am in Alpha Chi Omega sorority and am VP of fraternity relations. I am also the public relations rep for the University Hall executive board. I have a lot going on! Right now, I am trying really hard to study for my first round of college finals!

"My goals have changed some since I was ten years old," Katie says about her pretransplant take on the future. "When I was 10, I thought I could live to be 100 years old. I already wanted to go to college. I thought I'd maybe become a doctor, but I wasn't really sure. I was pretty certain I would want to work in a hospital. But I also thought about being a model! Now I'm studying communications with a concentration in public relations. I want to work for an organ bank, such as ROBI (Regional Organ Bank of Illinois). I want to work to educate the public, to talk to high school students about the need for organ donation. I want to help teens change their point of view regarding donation, to help them see its importance.

"I've never asked the doctor if I should have children of my own. I think I could carry a pregnancy, but I also think all the medications I am on might be bad for the baby. Also, I wouldn't want to have a child and then not be here for it. That's another difference between asking me this at 10 and at 18. At 10 years old I thought some day I'd have five babies!

As for right now, "I'm in good health. I'm at a good weight. At my six-month checkup my prednisone dose was decreased,

As recently as January 2004, MTV's reality show *Real World: San Diego* featured a college girl who had cystic fibrosis.

so my puffy cheeks started to go down. It'll take a full year before I can be on the lowest dose of prednisone, which is 10 mg. Then I'll be okay, and my cheeks will be back to normal. For now, I am just so happy that I can walk to the mall, bike, treadmill, and do weights without getting tired."

—Katie Kocelko

ANOTHER BOOK WORTH READING

Cystic Fibrosis in the 20th Century: People, Events, and Progress, edited by Carl F. Doershuk (Guilford, UK: AM Publishing, Ltd., 2002) chronicles the remarkable increase in survival and quality of life seen since the description of the disease in 1938, with memoirs that date back to the 1940s, history of the CF Foundation, medical advances, and much more.

A HARD DECISION: TO TRANSPLANT OR NOT

Another young lady, April, had a double lung transplant in January 2001.

"I was diagnosed with CF when I was going on 2 years old. I now have cystic fibrosis–related diabetes (insulin dependent), I had a double lung transplant when I was 17, and I have osteoporosis due to transplant. I needed the transplant because my CF got so bad I was on continuous oxygen 24/7 and in the hospital so frequently for 'tune-ups.' I was in the hospital for two to three weeks a month for the whole year before I was transplanted. I was listed for twenty-three months, twenty-three long months. My life has changed so much since the transplant. I hardly ever go into the hospital anymore, and I can do so much that I couldn't do before. I can play basketball with friends, go to the beach, swim, and do a lot of things that require energy to do. Now, instead of doing four treatments a day, I take a bunch of pills. I take about fifteen different pills a day and only Albuterol treatments when needed. Or, if I have an infection, sometimes I go on inhaled antibiotics. But that's about all for medicine. Well, I am also still on insulin. But since the transplant, my diabetes has done so much better now, too."—April Harris-Kinsey, 20, Englewood, Florida

Lung transplant is not the right option for everyone. Some are too sick, and others feel it's not what they want for themselves. Ultimately, when it comes to making the decision to have a transplant, the decision is your own. It takes a great deal of strength and courage to decide to have a transplant. It takes a great deal of strength and courage to decide *not* to have a transplant, too.

"I'm not interested in a lung transplant. My mom wants me to find out about it but said she won't make me do it. I don't want to be cut open. I don't want the process. If they could just go, 'Boom! There are your new lungs!' I'd be fine. But I don't want the, 'What's your weight? What's your blood pressure?' All that beforehand for a few months and then the transplant and then having to recuperate and then wondering if my body is going to take them or reject them. It's not that I don't have time for all that. I say I don't have time . . . but I have plenty of time to do all that. But I don't want to.

"I'm sicker than I say. I know I'm sick, and I know that my lungs are probably in bad condition. I know that I'm sicker than I want to admit, but if I say, 'I'm sick, I'm sick, I have CF, I can't do this,' then I'll never get to do the things I want to do. So I try to say, 'No, no, I'm healthy.' I go and I go. I think it's psychological. I'm sure sooner or later I'm going to die, too, like the rest [of my friends who had CF]. The way I see it, I'm living every day as it goes by, and I'm having a good time. And we all die. So I'm just going to die a little sooner than most.

Maybe it hasn't hit home yet, but I'm not bothered by it because when I die, how am I going to know that I could have had twenty more years of a good life if I'm dead? It's like, I won't know what I'm missing because I'll be gone."
—Kimberlee Pilarczyk, 20

Kimberlee died on May 11, 1996, eight days after celebrating her 21st birthday.

NOTES

1. Norma Kennedy Plourde's Cystic Fibrosis website, personal.nbnet.nb.ca/nnormap/CF.htm or www3.nbnet.nb.ca/normap/cfhistory.htm.
2. Diana K. Sugg, "The Famous Dead Yield Only Murky Diagnosis," *The Sun*, November 17, 2002, www.pulitzer.org/year/2003/beat-reporting/works/sugg6.html; and Kent State University, "What Killed Chopin," WKSU, www.wksu.org/classical/articles/what_killed_chopin.html.

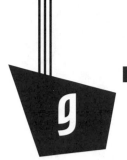

In the End

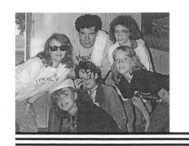

Six weeks into my freshman year of college . . . fifteen minutes until French class: I grabbed today's mail from my mailbox in the dorm lobby. I had several letters to open, which was exciting. Letters from home were always a treat for those away at college, especially in the days before e-mail. On one envelope, I recognized the return address as that of my new camp friend, Troy. I had spent a bit of extra time with Troy after camp because he had been admitted to Children's Memorial Hospital several times over the summer. We'd shared ice cream and pizza, and I'd even brought my sister and a couple of friends up to his room to meet this brave and amazing boy. Not quite 15 years old, Troy was a small boy, younger looking than his peers, but a Romeo with a big heart and a teddy-bear-soft haircut. All of the girls his age had crushes on him. Three years his senior, I adored him for who he was and for the friendship we had built so quickly. How happy I was to receive a letter from him. I ripped at the envelope as I walked through the quad. The letter was not from Troy. It was from his mother. "Troy is dying," it began. My tears began to fall unchecked, and I went numb almost immediately. What should I do? How could I get to him in time? I stood still on the path that led through campus to my French class. I can't remember whether I actually made it to class that day or not. Sometime later I called home from my dorm room. I don't remember to whom I spoke. My sister, my father? I instructed someone in my family on what things to bring to Troy in the hospital, and I dictated a letter to him.

My sister called me back the next day. "He looked so skinny," she told me after she had made my deliveries. She was just a few months older than Troy. Her future was so bright, so much different from Troy's. "Skinnier even than he was this summer," she said, quietly, having only an idea of the full ramifications of her words.

A few of my new college friends came by on Sunday evening. We watched television together. I was thinking about nothing in particular except the fun weekend I had just had and how much I was really starting to enjoy college life. The phone rang. I reached for it without taking my eyes from the television and whatever show we happened to be watching. "Troy died today," his mother told me, describing how they had brought him home from the hospital so he could die. "Oh!—I'm so sorry!" were the words that made it out of my mouth, caught and saved quickly from the words that had first started to form, "Oh! My God!" I held back my tears while I listened to this brave woman tell me about her son, her little boy, my friend. I was devastated. My world seemed to crumble around me. I lost several hours that evening as I sat with one new friend, a guy from the first floor named Bob, and I tried as hard as I could to block out the crushing pain inside me. I lost a dear and special friend that night. One who, in his life and in his death, would ultimately change my life. I also gained several new friends at college that night, all of whom grew up just a little bit beside me as they helped me through some of the roughest moments of my life up to that point. It was September 26, 1986. Troy would have been 15 years old in a few weeks. It was the first time I would lose a friend to cystic fibrosis—but it would not be the last.

We come to a stop and I'm asked, "Are you ready?"
My head swings from side to side as I reach into the
    paper for the
Rose
The walk is forced, I feel almost dragged, and then
    we're there
I'm hit in the face—one strong blow knocks the tears
    from my eyes
We stand for a few minutes that seem to be 10 but are
    really 25
Two children too young to be here
The girl's hair blows blonde streaks across her face
The boy lights up a cigarette, and the girl says nothing
It's a nice spot, sun-drenched in the late fall afternoon
Just west of a young tree that provides shade in the
    early hours
He has no family with him here, save a neighbor, his
    grandfather
Who arrived several years before
He's here, just six feet below my new shoes, yet I
    can't touch
Him, much less believe what I know to be true
We wrap our arms around each other
The pain never ends
Neither does the love
Tears run free, but sobs are stifled
I think he'd want us to smile
"I remember the time, when I'd first met him . . ."
We smile
Our eyes remain fixed on the name, and the dates that
    are too close
Together
He was just a baby!
And it already seems so long ago
He hears the car horn, so I check my watch

(continued)

177

"Are you ready?" I'm asked again, only this time for
    the
Departure
I'm here now, but if I leave
Will I really believe that we were actually
Here now? A time to savor . . .
I press the yet unopened bud of the red rose to my
    lips—a kiss, my love
Just like the one I gave him right before . . .
He watches, I think, as I lay it down above his name
My fingers
Play
Briefly, lightly across that which is left—a name
Goodbye, again
He takes my hand and leads me blindly through tears
Across the grass
Leaving behind what we know is forever in our hearts.
—Melanie Ann Apel, 22, October 1, 1990

The scenario would repeat itself, at least in outcome, twice more during my college years. In the Septembers of my sophomore and senior years, I would say goodbye to my friends Angela Dibbern (in 1987) and Cris Shadle (in 1989). I came to expect it. My college friends also grew to expect this part of my life. And while it never became any easier, I—we—learned to cope with it better. I also learned to hate—and anticipate with dread—the month of September.

August, September
August
Begins to slide
To a close
Kids shop for school clothes
And notebooks

(continued)

I can feel
September
Whispering
Closely, just around the edges
Of my world
Tip-toeing closer
Trying to catch a grip
I can feel
Death
All around me
Closing in
And I wonder what I'll wear
And to whose . . .
Songs on the tape
And conversations
Bring it all so
Close—
The heartwarming past
The imminent future
The life-blossoming
The breath—struggling tenaciously to hold on
The death—the inevitable
That visits the night
To warn that September
Is ready again
Play the music, see the photos
Reminisce—and be
Grateful
For the gift of friendship
And the gift of
Precious
Life.
—Melanie Ann Apel, 22, August 26, 1990

"END-STAGE" CYSTIC FIBROSIS

In the end, things start to look bad. When a person who has cystic fibrosis gets close to the end of his or her life, he or she is said to have "end-stage cystic fibrosis." Quite a bit of lung damage has been sustained, despite all efforts via nebulizers, IVs, bronchial drainage, exercise, enzymes, feeding tubes, and hospitalizations. It's simply not enough. Cystic fibrosis is bigger than all the therapies and treatments combined. The end is near, though the will to fight will often linger just a bit longer.

The profile of someone who has end-stage CF looks like this: He or she has been on supplemental oxygen for a while, probably a year or so, first only at night, but now all the time. He or she is very thin, for despite the assistance of enzymes, it's simply impossible to take in enough calories to fight the shortness of breath that becomes a constant companion. It has become difficult to walk up stairs, or even to walk at all, and a wheelchair might become desirable for longer jaunts. Hospital stays increase in frequency and length and are often so unbalanced that the person is actually in the hospital more than out. School or work could be put on the back burner while all efforts are concentrated toward day-to-day health. At home, the regimen of breathing treatments and therapy sessions could be increased to four or more per day in an attempt to clear the damaged lungs for maddeningly shorter and shorter periods of time. High fevers, lung pain, hemoptysis, exhaustion, headaches, and depression, among other symptoms, could become frequent companions. Finally, the lungs are damaged beyond repair, they have lost their elasticity, they are filled with infection and mucus, and the person is no longer able to draw breath.

Not all of these things happen to everyone who dies of cystic fibrosis. Some people have other complications that get the best of them before any of these symptoms have a chance to set in. Others are able to maintain their weight while their lung function deteriorates. And still others succumb quickly to an infection that they were unable to shake. Regardless, the end sounds so painful and frightening. It is no wonder then that those who have CF fight hard to stay as healthy as possible for as long as possible. This is also the reason why it is so urgent that a cure be found.

Now approaching her 40th birthday, Cathy Carnevale has beaten the odds and lived long past the life expectancy for someone born with cystic fibrosis in the early 1960s. Cathy continues to face the challenges of cystic fibrosis every day. In a poignant letter just after we learned that our friend Angela Budnieski's life had been taken by complications of CF, Cathy wrote to me:

The visualization I get of the description we read in Angela's mom's letter is understandably horrifying. I just cannot (don't want to) picture that dying woman on failing life support as our little, dark-haired, smiling-faced, giggling Angela. I still remember her face vividly, and some of the letters she wrote to me for a while after camp. Forgive me for swearing, but damn this disease! Not for me, because I feel no pity for myself for having it, never really have—I've led a full life in spite of it. The anger I feel is over the cruel way in which it manifests itself and takes the innocents. I'm sure you'd agree that perhaps our first graphic description of the disease's ravaging was in Frank Deford's description of Alex's last moments. Because of that, I can imagine the same difficult end for my sister Clare, for Angela Dibbern, for Cris [Shadle], for the DiBiases, Lisa [Zepeda], Fonda [Langston], and on and on and *on*. I have to tell you, I had a very depressing day today, notwithstanding any thoughts of CF, and I'll admit further that it's days like today that I don't consider myself "lucky" to still be among the survivors of CF, when all those wonderful people we knew never got the chance to live this long. Yes, I'm feeling bitter right now. Bitter that they were taken from this world, and from our lives, and so painfully, in so many cases. And *yes*, even bitter to have been left behind to endure the continued pain of seeing more and more of them go to that wonderful camp in the sky where they can run and swim and stay up all night talking and laughing and not have to take hundreds of pills and hours of treatments anymore just to breathe and feel good . . .
Love, Cathy

You can read about cystic fibrosis in books and on the Internet, and you might know others who are living with CF with whom you can share stories and exchange anecdotes, but no one can really tell you how your life will play out if you have CF. And this fact can be frightening. While the official statistics state 35.1 years as the median life span for someone who has CF, there are no guarantees. No one, not even your doctor, can accurately predict that you will live to be 35. There is no guarantee that you won't fly past 35 and live for many more years, either.

"I am a 36-year-old woman with cystic fibrosis," says Jo-Anne Giles of Western Australia. Already three years past the "median age" of life expectancy, Jo-Anne says, "I have experienced a serious decline in my health since I've hit 30. I was born in 1968 and the prognosis was not good for us back then. We were not expected to reach adulthood. Advances in medical research, advances we could not have even dreamt of, have made it possible for the majority of us to reach adulthood."

Fear of the unknown can be hard to come to grips with. Yet, everyone lives with the unknown, whether you have CF or not. Just like healthy people, anyone can die in an accident or succumb to some other type of illness, such as cancer. There are no certainties. Just as there is no "typical" case of CF.

Some people who have CF deal with difficulties all their lives. Others—those with milder cases—live relatively "normal" lives by comparison. It might actually be more

Did You Know?
Former CBS television football analyst Jimmy "the Greek" Snyder (1918–1996) had two sons who had CF.[1]

Each May, the Cystic Fibrosis Foundation hosts its largest national event, the Great Strides: Taking Steps to Cure Cystic Fibrosis ten kilometer walk. Find out about the 550 walk sites across the country by visiting www.cff.org/great_strides.

difficult for the healthier person to come to grips with CF as he or she gets older and begins to feel the effects of CF on his or her body. The person who has been sick all his or her life might be more accustomed to the disease and its challenges.

Whether your CF has been relatively easy to deal with or has caused you trouble all your life, as you get older you are likely to experience more and more physical difficulties. You might find yourself in the hospital more frequently. You might have to take more medications to achieve the same results you were once able to achieve with less effort. You might feel tired more often, have less energy and less strength, or not feel quite "yourself." Some people who have CF mention that they have increased pain when they are breathing, or they cough up blood more often (although not everyone who has CF coughs up blood). You might even begin to feel less and less as if you are in control of your disease; you might begin to feel as if your disease is controlling you. It will become harder and harder than usual to shake illnesses such as colds and the flu. The inevitable progression of cystic fibrosis can be very frightening.

When it comes to taking good care of yourself, some might say, "Why bother?" Many would agree, however, that it's the quality of life that counts rather than the quantity. In order to provide the best quality of life, healthcare providers prescribe the full regime of available medications and therapies. Always have hope!

While some people opt for and receive lung transplants, some die waiting for suitable donor lungs (the current average wait time on the transplant list is twenty months), and still others decide not

> "Following Troy's and Angela's deaths, I had to work on my reaction so as not to shut my own world down. I was doing fairly well until my friend Jenny DiBiase died on June 24, 1994."—Melanie Ann Apel

to have the surgery at all. The sad reality about cystic fibrosis is that in the end, sometimes sooner and sometimes later, it's always fatal. And it's always heartbreaking.

KEN, THE BROTHER WITHOUT CF

In a very articulate and poignant interview taped fifteen months after his 22-year-old sister Jenny lost her battle with cystic fibrosis, Ken DiBiase described life as the healthy brother of two siblings with CF. Still trying to cope with Jenny's death at the time, Ken was faced with the reality of his brother Mike's pending death. Ken was raw with emotion as he discussed the impact of Mike and Jenny's lives on his own.

"I don't remember a time without CF," begins Ken in a 1995 interview. Ken is seated in a waiting room at Children's Memorial Hospital in Chicago, where his brother Mike is a patient. "My brother Mike is only two years younger than me, and I was too young to remember when he was diagnosed." In fact, Ken realizes, "I think Jenny was diagnosed first. Mike was two when Jenny was born. They diagnosed Jenny, and then they decided to check Mike and me. Mike ended up having CF, while I did not. CF was always just there. It was normal. I knew I didn't have CF. When we were young, Mike and Jenny really weren't much different from me because, before they started getting sick, they could do pretty much anything I could do. Mike played basketball and Jenny used to run and play. Life was pretty normal for us as little kids. The only difference I can remember at that point was that they had to take their enzyme pills everyday and I didn't. But I never felt different. The first time Mike went into the hospital, I think it was 1980, was the first time CF ever really manifested itself, and I really noticed it. After that, the hospital stays became more routine because both Mike and Jenny would go in once or twice a year. They would stay for their ten or fourteen days and get 'cleaned out' or 'tuned up' as everyone called it. Then they would come back home, and we'd have our normal life with just these little interruptions. Life stayed fairly normal for at least ten years or so. I moved to California, leaving my family behind in Illinois, so I didn't really see how bad things were getting.

"Jenny was really sick. I had no idea," Ken says, remembering back to June of 1994. "I only knew when Mike called me the night before; that's when I finally knew how bad it was. As I recall his exact words were, 'You'd better come here.' I made my plane reservation and took a 6:30 a.m. flight

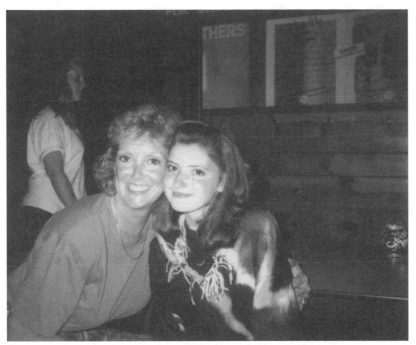

Jenny DiBiase and one of her favorite respiratory therapists, Paula Mowbray, at CF camp.

back to Chicago. I saw her and talked to her. I don't even know if she heard me or saw me. She must have," Ken reflects, "because she died a few hours after I got there.

"I had known she was in the hospital of course, but from the way my parents and even Mike had talked to me, we all thought she would be released, as usual. This stay was probably a little less routine, but we never thought her death was imminent, until Mike said she took this horrible turn for the worse one night. And that's when they knew. They called me about two days after that and told me to come home. I knew it up here in my head, but I didn't know it down here," Ken says, tapping lightly on his chest, over his own heart. "There was no way to prepare for it."

"I've always been told that most CF patients don't live past 20. Jenny was 22. In the past few years, I had always kind of thought in the back of my mind that it could happen in a few years, you know, in five years. But thinking about it intellectually does not prepare you for it emotionally.

"When Jenny died, I cried a lot. Everyone was a wreck, really. Our family stayed together for a long time in the hospital. My cousin and our childhood friends from the old neighborhood were there. It was just like the old group back from when we were kids. The emotional support of having all those people there helped."

At this point, Ken recognizes the fact that the health of his younger brother Mike, who is 25 years old, is declining. Having just brought Mike to the hospital to be admitted, Ken now sees firsthand how bad things are for his brother. "I think it is definitely not easier. If anything, it's a lot harder. With Jenny, I wasn't here. I didn't know how bad it was. But now, with Mike, I am here. I do know how bad it is.

"Mike's doctors seem to think his only hope is to have a lung transplant. So right now I am just thinking about that transplant. I am sure he is thinking about it, too. We've pinned all our hopes on it, but really that is what it is. It needs to happen very soon. His lungs will never get better. I'll respect his decision if he decides not to have the transplant, though. I would have to. Then I would have to prepare myself because I know what would happen next. I've told him what I think, but ultimately it's his decision. I told him that I can't imagine how he feels because I don't know what it's like not to be able to breathe or take a shower because it's too much effort, or walk upstairs, or ride a bike, or run. There are pros and cons to this operation, and I told him that the pros are that he would be able to do all of these things and more without getting out of breath.

"Mike is declining. I can see a difference since last I saw him three months ago. He was tired then, but not as bad as he is now. One thing I remember about Jenny in the later stages was that it was always so hard for her to take a shower. I couldn't understand that. Like, showering is not that hard. But I guess when you can hardly breathe, it is. Mike says it's hard for him now to take a shower. That's when it finally hit me, like wow! Showering is something we take for granted: we hop in, we hop out. So this was a big alarm going off in my head.

"I think Mike wants to live. But he has different religious beliefs than I do, and he says that if it's meant to be, it will be. I think we have choices; we can change things. He can decide to have the transplant in hopes of saving his own life. He doesn't have to just accept death. I think that's what he'll do. I hope that's what he'll do." Ken thinks about his family's reaction to

Jenny's death and wonders what would happen in the event that Mike doesn't make it.

"Mike and Christin (their then-19-year-old sister) have become much closer since Jenny died. Christin is really frantic about Mike's health now. I thought Christin dealt with Jenny's death really well. I was impressed with her composure. Both my parents were devastated. I think my dad handled it the worst. He wanted nothing to do with making the funeral arrangements. Mike and my mom and I took care of everything. I think it helped my mom to keep busy.

"I don't think they think about Mike dying. Like maybe if they don't think about it, it will go away or even get better. Maybe they do think about it.

"If I could change things, go back to the beginning when we were all little; well, I'm going to state the obvious: I would change the fact that they had CF. I'm selfish, I know that if Jenny hadn't had CF she would still be here, and I still want her here. I don't know what her life would be like now, at 23, if she were alive and didn't have CF. She'd probably be working, just leading a normal life. She'd probably have her own place, maybe here in the city. I don't know if she'd be married by now, but I'm sure she'd be dating. That's one of the worst, saddest things; Jenny never really had a boyfriend. I mean she did, I guess, like at camp and stuff, but no one who came to the house and that she dated for a long time exclusively because she was sick all the time. But, I'm sure if she were alive and healthy, she would be dating because she was very pretty and very nice."

Ken thinks about his own life and his future. Although he does not plan to have children of his own, he feels that if he were in a position to have a family, he wouldn't let CF stop him. "I don't know if I am a CF carrier or not, but if I wanted to have kids, I wouldn't let that stand in my way. I would want to have them whether they had CF or not.

"The best thing about having Mike and Jenny as my siblings is being exposed to their personalities. Mike is always really optimistic, in spite of hardships and everything. Jenny was always laughing. They're always happy and optimistic despite their difficulties. They make me feel good. The worst thing is seeing them sick, and then feeling like it didn't have to be this way. They could have been born healthy and things would have been so much different. If only this didn't happen. It's a feeling of frustration, I guess. That crosses my mind a lot, the 'why did this have to happen?' And if I were a really religious person, I would be railing at God. But I am not religious, so I just have this frustration that I don't know what to do with. I just accept it as best as I can. It's just genetics. I don't sit and stew over it, but sometimes I think it would have been nice to dance with Jenny or play tennis with Mike.

"I have accepted Jenny's death, intellectually, at least. It's weird because sometimes I just think she's on a really long vacation, and she'll be coming back soon. But I know she won't. I don't think there was ever a point when I felt relieved, like, well that's over. Things got easier when I got back to California, but I think it's a long, continuous process.

"A lot of my friends don't understand CF at all. I try to explain it as best as I can, but they are really confused most of the time. They don't hear about CF as much as some other diseases or disorders. There are many facets to the disease that I am still realizing even now. I thought it was just that they have trouble breathing and they can't digest food. But then so many other things crop up; like, I didn't know how badly affected they are by a simple cold.

"I dream about Jenny a lot. It's kind of neat. Half the time I dream about her when she was sick, and a lot of times I dream about her healthy. Those are weird. It's like, wow, so this is what she would have looked like! It feels good to wake up from those dreams, as if she were still really here with me in a way. It's like I got to see her again and it's the only way I know how to see her, other than in photos. I don't dream about her every night, maybe only a few times a month. I definitely miss her a lot. I miss her laugh the most. I can still hear Jenny laugh. She had an infectious laugh. I loved that. She was so funny. She always made me laugh with the things she would say out of nowhere. She would imitate people, like my mom or my aunt, and she would be dead-on accurate. I just had to laugh. It's harder for Mike to laugh now because he always ends up coughing. He was smiling a lot last night though when our friend Ed was here. We were joking around a lot. He was in pretty good spirits I would have to say. His sense of humor is much drier than Jenny's was. He's more sarcastic, and his sarcasm is hilarious. I don't even know if I have a sense of humor. My humor is more on the cynical side probably.

"Another thing I remember about her was that she was meticulous about her appearance. She was very attentive to her nails and her hair. She always wanted to look nice. I think she had a great sense of style. She was very much a lady. I think Jenny taught Christin a lot, too. They might have bickered and fought a lot, but deep down they had a bond because they were sisters. Jenny cared deeply about people. She was always telling me to be careful when I went out and stuff like that. She always wanted to make sure everyone was okay.

"Mike is the kind of person who would do anything for you. I just think how great it would be if Mike got the transplant and it's successful. Things would be so different for him, like night and day."—Ken DiBiase, 27

Jenny DiBiase and I got to know each other and became friends during the week of CF camp 1990. I knew I was setting myself up; I knew I was taking a risk getting to know Jenny. I knew we could become close, we would become attached, we would find a love in our friendship, and then I would lose. I knew that sooner or later, and probably sooner rather than later, Jenny would die, and as her friend, my heart would break. And it did. Every day for a week I watched helplessly from Jenny's bedside as she lost more and more ground. I cried at home and in the car, as God seemed to be doing as well. It rained all week. And then on Friday, late in the afternoon, the clouds slipped aside to allow bright sunshine to slip through. I knew that Jenny was free.

LOSING JENNY: MIKE'S STORY

Shortly after the interview with Ken DiBiase, his younger brother Mike was released from Children's Memorial Hospital. On full-time supplemental oxygen, Mike knew that a lung transplant was his only chance. Yet his faith in God and his love and devotion for his sister Jenny eased his fear of death. Mike contemplated Jenny's life and his own, while offering another perspective of life in the DiBiase family.

"Back at the beginning, when we were younger, CF was not any big deal to us. All it meant to Jenny and me was that we had to take a couple of pills when we ate and go to the clinic every few months. That's really it. We lived totally normal lives. We never had any bad lung infections or any hospitalizations when we were real young. We didn't even get therapy at home. My parents did it for awhile, but we wouldn't want to sit down and get pounded. We were too busy running around playing. We weren't really too affected.

"The first time I was in the hospital was when I was ten years old. I got really sick with a lung infection at camp. I don't remember—even as I'm getting sicker now—feeling worse than I did then. I could barely take two steps, maybe ten at the most. My lips and nails were blue. I just could not breathe. That might have been when I was initially infected with *pseudomonas.*

"Jenny was in the hospital for the first time the same year. She was 8. From that point we went in occasionally. It started out maybe once every couple of years and then maybe once a year. In my adolescent years, I had long breaks before I had to go in the hospital. Probably because I was still pretty active. Then the hospitalizations grew increasingly shorter apart there for awhile. As I got into my 20s, I would forcefully try to make it longer between hospitalizations even though I probably should have been going in more frequently. Jenny went in more frequently than I did because she didn't have any stubbornness about it. Actually, there were times when Jenny went in less frequently than I did, between the ages of 10 and 15, simply because I think she was much healthier than I was. But later on when we both needed to go in about the same amount, I would stick it out and try not to go even though I should have. She would be more diligent than I was and go in and do what she had to do, get the antibiotics, and then be out of there. She did what she had to do in terms of her health.

"I started working for my uncle when I was 20 and that helped a lot. It kept me active and kept me to where I had enough physical activity so that my lungs stayed somewhat healthy. When Jenny started going into the hospital more, I started to take care of her more than my parents did because Jenny and I started to get real close. A couple factors were involved: our shared faith in God and the fact that we could relate to the disease. Jenny and I started to become real close, and basically I did everything for her. I would take her to the clinics, the doctor, and the hospital. Usually when she was in the hospital, I would stay with her most of the time. My parents would visit. But since I was there to do those things it freed my parents up. I don't know if deep down they didn't realize that she was getting as sick as she was, or if it was just too hard for them to deal with it. But I kind of stepped up to the plate and really took care of her in her later years.

"When she died, it was a little surprising for me. I knew she was getting sicker, but I thought she might have a few months left or something like that. It wasn't really clear to me that this was going to be her last hospitalization, even though she was pretty sick. When I look back . . . hindsight is always twenty/twenty. I can see it and I'm like, how could I have not seen it? But to me that's not a big deal because I don't have any regrets. I loved her as much as I possibly could. Sometimes people look back with a bunch of regrets and say, 'I wish I could have done this . . .' but our relationship was strong.

"I met Dr. Wessel once in the elevator and he said to me, 'What does she feel about dying?' And I said, 'She knows that she's sick enough that she could die. She can accept that.' He said, 'Well, ok.'

"But see, he had said that to me a couple times before when she had been sick, too. Like within the last year when she had been going downhill he would say that to me. So I really didn't think of this last time as any different than before. No one really said, 'She's going to die.' I don't know if people really expected it to happen, like if the nurses really thought that she was going to die during this admission, or if the doctors thought just that things could take a turn for the worse. I've had a lot of experience seeing kids on their deathbeds, in terms of CF, going in and saying good-bye to them. Jenny wasn't yet in that state where she was fighting to breathe, so I didn't think that. . . . I thought it would be a slower process than the way it actually was. When she finally did take the turn for the worse, it was instantaneous. The respiratory therapist came in at five-thirty on Thursday morning to give her a treatment because she wanted them more frequently. All of a sudden her mind just kind of freaked out. While the therapist was giving her the treatment she said, 'Where's my therapist? I need a treatment. Go get my therapist.' She had the nebulizer in her mouth, and he was pounding on her. When he was done he said, 'OK, you can go back to sleep now.' And she just sat there, and she looked at him and said, 'Can you go get my therapist? I need a treatment.' So her mind was kind of acting funny. That was the morning she just kind of went out of it. She was out of it for that whole day. I don't think she had a problem concentrating before that point.

"You [the author] came for a visit, and you'd written a card for Jenny. Jenny just stared blankly at it for a few minutes before she handed the card back and said, 'Here, you can read this for me; I can't see straight.' I didn't know that this meant she was close to the end. A couple of nights before that we were playing cards. She was like, 'How do you play this game?' And it was some game that she had taught me. She couldn't play the game. She would put down funny cards for rummy. It would be just a bunch of different cards that meant nothing. But I didn't know that meant that she could go into that coma state or whatever you'd call it.

"She was like this all day Thursday and most of Friday until she died.

"I know I keep saying this, but I didn't really think she was going to die. I knew she was sick, but I thought that she was . . . because she was going through the process for a transplant . . . so I thought. . . . I was still hoping that she would get through what she needed to do to get on the list before she got out of the hospital. I think there's that hope that keeps you from really seeing reality sometimes. You're hoping and hoping and hoping, so you're not really trying to focus on the negative.

"The last admission, when she died, she was just in for the same thing she had always gone in for, although, actually, she was coughing up more blood. But it just seemed like the same kind of hospitalization she had had the last few times, where she would go in and get her treatments and come home. The last few times she would never get better during the hospitalization. She wasn't getting better, but they were keeping her kind of stable enough, just kind of buying time so she could get on the transplant list.

"I guess maybe I didn't see it because Jenny had gotten to the point where she kind of lay around anyway. That's probably why I didn't notice what was really taking place. At home all she ever really did was lie around. That's basically all she did for the last few months. She had been on oxygen since September. She really didn't do much. She didn't really go out. Her friends didn't really come over.

"That's how we're different, because I've made it a point to get out every day since I've gotten home from the hospital. I've made sure to get a little bit of exercise, even if it's just getting out and driving around. Because I know that once you're on oxygen, you have to keep yourself ventilating pretty well; otherwise, your CO_2 is just going to build up and build up. Jenny didn't do this. She didn't know. I didn't know either. I learned through Jenny, what Jenny went through. I can see the signs taking place in my life now—the degrees of the disease. I'm obviously not doing great, but I'm not to the point where I'm bedridden, so I try to make the best of it.

"I don't think Jenny gave up. She still did her treatments every day, even when she didn't do anything and just sat around all day. Plus, she was doing her Vest a little bit, but mainly I did her therapy. But there's no handbook that gives you directions [for] how to react to each particular instance when your health starts going down. If she had given up, I know she wouldn't have been doing those things. She did them every day, religiously. There's this kind of blind ignorance that people can get with CF. I know I was getting it. You don't really realize how bad you're getting because it's a slow, progressive thing. It's like, if you watch a child grow up and you're the parent, you don't really notice how much they've changed. But to someone who hasn't seen the child in a long time, they can say, 'Wow! Your child has really changed. He's growing up.' That's kind of what it is like with CF. While you're living every day with it, you're progressively getting worse, but I don't think you really notice it to a great degree.

"I think Jenny knew that she could die. But I don't think that she knew she was actually going to die when she did. I think she had hopes of being around, and she decided that she wanted to do the transplant. I know she was trying to hang on to the hopes of beating this thing because there's been so much talk about the cure and the gene therapy. In her head, I think that she was trying to hold out strong [so] that maybe she could partake in that. But it got to the point where she finally sat there and said, ok, I'll do the transplant, because she realized that [gene therapy] wasn't a reality anymore. Really deep down maybe she knew she was going to die, but I never saw any evidence of it.

"CF was something she could look right in the face. She was genuinely not afraid of dying. For a long time we would talk about dying; we would talk to each other about how if I would ever die, she would make sure that this or that was done, and I would say, 'If you ever die, I'd make sure that this or that was done.' Her faith was very strong. She believed that the Lord would take care of her. Once she put her faith in the Lord, it wasn't a matter of her having to perform, to make sure the good outweighed the bad in her life.

"She had told me she had been writing some things down in her journal, but I didn't know what it was; I had never read it. Jenny's writing allowed just a glimpse into her heart. The day I came home from the hospital after she died things were really rough. The first thing I did was see if I could find her journal. I wanted to see what she had written. The things she said in there were actually deeper than I had even known she had experienced in terms of her relationship with God in her life. Like the things she said about talking with God. It was very encouraging to me because I know that she had a strong faith. Those excerpts from her journal were even more evidence to me. I was able to pick myself up and get through the next few days, through the wake and the funeral. That's just another way that she provided me with strength to just carry on.

"In terms of my brother, Ken, and my sister, Christin, growing up, I couldn't tell you whether they were jealous or not. I couldn't give you any evidence that they were. I don't know what my brother had to say about it, but I don't think there was any type of animosity or like, 'Oh they're getting all the attention.' Like I said, we didn't get excess attention. We were normal, and we were dealt with just in the same way as my brother and sister were. I know Jenny didn't feel anything against them because they're healthy, and I can tell you I never have. I look at them, and I'm glad that they're healthy, even when I get impatient with my brother, and I lash out at him or get angry. There are times when my brother, more than my sister, is not very understanding about the disease. You know, he's kind of clueless sometimes. He's very impatient in some ways. He gets angry very easily at some things. Like, if I'm sick and he's walking around getting mad about the simple things in life, and I'm sitting there with a really bad lung infection. Sometimes, I would like to shake him and say, 'Ken, your problems are not that rough. Look at Jenny; she went through this whole thing, and she never got mad at everybody.'

Sometimes, like recently, if I were getting out of breath, he would try to push me, like, 'Well, come on; can you hurry up a little?' When you can't breathe and you have someone trying to tell you to hurry up, you want to just say, 'Shut up, alright?' But I thought about it, and I remember myself saying to him, 'Maybe one day you'll know how it feels.' But really, in all sincerity, I hope that he never has to know because it's not something I would wish on anybody. I would wish that people would just have good health. So, a couple times I've caught myself being angry and saying something like that, like, 'Maybe one day you'll know. . . .' I've never said, 'I hope some day you'll know . . .' because I hope that he doesn't ever have to know. I just try to get more patient with him sometimes.

"He's come around a lot. He's different now than he was growing up. He's much more helpful now, maybe because he was forced to be. He's been much more helpful in the last year since Jenny died. He's been more understanding, probably because he realizes how serious CF is. I didn't even realize how serious it was until recently. I still don't realize. It's a defense mechanism maybe, I don't know. That's what we thought, though, that it couldn't possibly really happen. You don't want to believe that you're getting as sick as you are. I've heard so many cystics say it. I've said it to myself. How many times have you heard this? 'I'm not as sick as they are.' In reality there are a lot of cystics who are just as sick as the next. In a way sometimes, that's a good thing because that's what's going to keep their will to live driving. Like who's that girl who just died? Lisa Cochran. She was Jenny's roommate. She had a collapsed lung, and she couldn't even walk around. She sounded terrible, and at that time Jenny was much healthier than she, even though Jenny was thinner. I shouldn't say much healthier, but she was a little bit healthier. I remember Lisa Cochran saying, 'But see, I'm not as sick as *most* cystics.' And I remember thinking, 'But you are.' I realized that I was just as guilty of that type of mentality too. Later on, I said the same thing, 'I'm not as sick as . . .' or, 'I'll never get like that.' All cystics are going to think that. That's just part of the process. So I had, I don't know what you want to call it, denial or whatever. You just believe that you're never going to get that sick.

"I talked to Mike Williams yesterday. I shouldn't make a judgment, but on the phone his voice sounded terrible, he sounded really junky. Maybe he was just having a bad day. He was talking like he was not that bad, and I was thinking to myself, 'I hope you're not that bad! But you don't really sound that good.' But am I right in that? I've seen cystics look at others and say, 'Boy I'm glad I'm not that bad,' or something like that. I remember in all the years at camp I always thought that. And then the reality hits you that people with CF, even the healthiest ones, are going to have to come to the point where they realize that they're sick. It's funny when you realize it because you realize you haven't been very nice. I mean, I could have probably spent more time with people who were sicker than I was at camp. I could have had more fun with people who couldn't run around and stuff. People have to grow up sometimes and realize those things. I don't think I even yet realize exactly how much I've learned. I think it will play itself out more, just in terms of being able to look at cystics and know what they're thinking and then know what it . . . feels like when somebody dies in your family; to know the pain of the initial loss and then just playing itself out and the short-term emotions and the long-term emotions.

"When Jenny died, the initial pain was hard. It was a real sadness. They always say that it gets better as time goes on. That's true except in the aspect of missing them a lot more over time. The sadness can go away, but that longing feeling to be with them just gets worse. It's just the feeling you get in your gut when you think of them. You know, like, if I could just give them a big hug just for one second—stuff like that. That doesn't go away like the sadness.

"Things were rather routine as far as end-stage CF goes when Jenny died. The condition I'm used to seeing with someone dying of CF is where they're just lying back and the bed is tilted up; they're sitting up, and they're just gasping for every breath. Every muscle in their neck is moving to help them breathe, and even their nostrils are flaring in an effort to grab more oxygen. You basically see every muscle in their upper body just moving to make them breathe. And they're out of it. They can't communicate to you. And they're pale. When I saw Jenny like that, that's when I knew she was going to die. That's just an irreversible condition. So I picked up the phone and called my mom and said, 'Mom, you need to come down to the hospital.' I didn't say she was going to die, even though I knew

it. I knew my mom knew it. I said, 'Things are bad.'
Fortunately my dad hadn't left for work yet. I told everyone to
come down to the hospital. My brother was in California, so he
got on a plane as soon as he could, which wasn't until the next
morning, so Jenny fought. She was out of it, but she knew
enough to know who was there, and I really believe that she
fought, and she was forcing herself to breathe until Ken came
the next day. He didn't get there till around one thirty or two
o'clock on Friday afternoon. Jenny died at about three o'clock.
He wasn't even there much more than an hour before she died.
She fought more than a day and a half. I kept telling her,
'Kenny's coming.' I wasn't saying, 'Hold on till you see Kenny,'
because I wouldn't want her to think that she had to try . . . it
wasn't like that. I just said, 'Kenny's coming to see you.' I kept
encouraging her that Kenny was on his way.

"Other people were coming in and out to see her. She would
have times where she would open her eyes, and she would come
out of it for brief moments. When Bridget, her best friend from
childhood, came in, she opened her eyes and said, 'Bridgy,
Bridge!' She kept calling her name and smiling almost as if she
saw her from her childhood or something, and she remembered
all that. Early on Thursday morning, my aunt had a baby girl,
and when we told her, Jenny opened her eyes and said, 'girl.'
That was kind of special. So I know that there were points in
time when she could hear us. That's why I kept telling her
Kenny was coming. And I would read her stuff from the Bible
that talked about going into glory and when you leave your
body and you're present with the Lord. The scripture talks
about there being no pain and no suffering, no tears, no crime,
no death. I was just trying to encourage her. I know she heard
me. On Friday, I was sitting there talking to her, and she opened
her eyes. She just kept saying, 'I love you, I love you.' That was
special because I think this was the last thing she said.

"Sometimes I feel bad that my parents didn't get an
opportunity to really talk with her before she went into that
state. But, I don't dwell on it too much because I know that
Jenny and I had a special relationship, a deeper relationship
than she had with my mom or dad, so it's not like she was
leaving them out.

"I remember when we were in her room and everyone was
around; we would wonder if she was in any pain or anything,

and we would ask her. The thought of giving her morphine had come up. I didn't want to give her any because I wanted her to be as coherent as possible in case she did want to say something to anybody. If there had been any evidence that she was in pain, I would have said go ahead with the morphine. We kept asking her, 'Are you in any pain? Are you in any pain?' And she would shake her head no. So I said, 'Ok, no medicine.' I was in charge of making decisions for the last couple of years. I look back, and I think if my parents would have known that she was dying, they would have taken a greater role in a lot of the stuff that happened. It's just that, like I said, there's a strange type of ignorance that can affect people so that they don't really see what's happening. A lot of times my parents thought the opposite of what was true. When Jenny got the feeding tube, they thought she was going to be healthier because she was getting the feedings. When she went on oxygen, they thought it was great because they thought she was going to be healthier because of it. But that wasn't the case. The feedings and the oxygen were because her body wasn't doing well, not because they were going to make her so much better.

"In the end what happened was this: We were all just coming and going. People would come and visit and sit with Jenny for awhile. Close friends and family. Genever from housekeeping came in. Jenny was giving her the thumbs up. That was awesome. I take a Christian perspective. I know that Genever has talked to me; she seems to be a strong Christian and Jenny was too. It was almost like Jenny was saying don't worry, you know, I'll see you on the other side. She knew Genever's inside spirit, and she knew she was seeing her for the final time. She could barely lift her arm and her thumb was like hanging there. But she was making the effort.

"On Friday, we were all on the bed right when Ken got there and that was it for Jenny. She had seen us all there together, and we had seen her. We were all there by the bedside, my mom, my dad, Christin, Kenny, and me; she opened her eyes, just for a moment, and she looked at Ken, and she looked back, and she closed her eyes. She saw Ken, but he didn't see her see him. That's why he kind of felt bad afterward. He was like, 'Do you think she even knew I was there?' And I said, 'She knew! I saw her.' I had seen her open her eyes. Ken had just gotten there; he was a little frazzled, and he wasn't really paying much attention. But I saw her; she looked up, and she saw him, and then she put her head back down. That was the last time she saw us really all together over the bed. Then people would sit down, maybe my mom would walk out, or my dad would walk out, but there was always someone by her bed at any given time.

"Then for some reason we had all left the room and we were in the lounge. I think her nurse was going to try to clean her up a little or lift her or something. We had just all stepped out for just a short minute, and then all of a sudden my cousin came running and she was saying, 'Quick the nurse said to come in.' The nurse was in there with my cousin Laura and her best friend Bridget. Samantha, the respiratory therapist, was in there too because Jenny's oxygen saturations were going really low. Samantha thought maybe Jenny's pulse ox (pulse oximeter: a device used to detect the amount of oxygen in the blood) lead had come off or something, but it hadn't. She had just started to go. And none of us were there when she died. We were all out of the room, and I think she did it that way because she didn't want to see or hear us crying or being sad while she was dying. She just wanted to remember us before. That can't be proven, but I say she just kind of slipped out the back door. And when we came in, she had stopped breathing. I heard noises coming from her chest, but it was more like air that was escaping. I just grabbed her and hugged her. My parents and everyone was crying. That was it. That was when she died. It was just about three o'clock in the afternoon on Friday, June 24, 1994.

"We sat around for a little bit in the lounge and in the room while the chaplain came up. It was so strange; it was like, after she initially died and people grieved for a certain amount of time, we were in the room and everything was like normal. Not normal—it's hard to describe. It wasn't like people were sobbing and sobbing for hours afterward. It was like, ok, she died. She had been at a point where she was breathing and struggling for so long that it was getting hard to watch her suffer like that. Obviously, she was fighting to breathe, and when she died, it was almost good to see that she was at rest."—Mike DiBiase

Late into 1996 Mike often asked, "Don't you think I should be getting my transplant soon? I've been waiting for awhile now." It wasn't a complaint about the time he was spending on the transplant list. It was just a matter of curiosity, paired with quiet desperation, as he felt himself growing sicker and weaker.

Finally, when he could no longer breathe on his own, Mike was placed on a ventilator as a last-ditch effort to hold out for a transplant. A set of donor lungs became available at the eleventh hour. Mike got his transplant in early November 1996. He was the first patient at his medical center harboring *Berkholderia cepacia* in his lungs to receive a transplant. He responded well and was able to go home after a couple of weeks. Mike died peacefully in his sleep one month after his transplant—eighteen months after his sister Jenny—on December 8, 1996, due to an abscess that developed between his heart and his lungs. He was 26 years old.

> **"One never recovers from such losses, but their sweet memories give us inspiration to help those who are determined to survive this insidious disease."**
> **—Hal Soloff, 73, Norwich, Connecticut**

NOTE

1. Norma Kennedy Plourde's Cystic Fibrosis website, personal.nbnet.nb.ca/nnormap/CF.htm or www3.nbnet.nb.ca/normap/cfhistory.htm.

Just over the Horizon

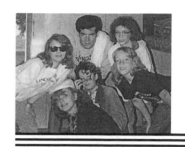

I had no idea where my years at CF camp would take me. As unfortunate as it was that many campers went into the hospital in the weeks immediately following camp each year, I loved the fact that I lived within walking distance from the hospital and could visit if summoned. And I visited often. It was fun. My non-CF friends thought I was crazy to want to hang out with kids at the hospital when I could be out at a party or doing something else. But we did all sorts of things during my visits. We rented movies, ordered pizza, and gathered in the teen lounge to talk. Back in the early days, the kids got passes to leave the hospital and go outside. So we went for walks or to the zoo, and a few times I even brought a small group back to my house for dinner. But things changed; soon patients were no longer allowed to leave on passes, and I thought about how great it would be to work daily with these amazing kids, many of whom were close to my own age. I enrolled in a respiratory therapy program at National-Louis University and become a respiratory therapist.

Over the next six years, I met all sorts of kids who had CF but who hadn't come to camp with us. And I became close friends with some of the younger campers whom I hadn't known as well at camp. Our camp's final year was 1993. It seems like ages ago, and in some ways CF is such a different disease now. But in the way that counts most—the way it continues to take my friends—it has not changed. Every August, when the *chill begins to creep back into the early mornings, I feel the breeze, I smell the dewy air, and I feel as if something important were missing: CF camp. I had said I would go until a cure was found and there was no more need for camp.*

In 1989 the future began to look brighter for those who have cystic fibrosis. As the 1980s drew to a close, researchers closed in on the gene that causes cystic fibrosis. The news made headlines: "CF Gene Found!"

In an article entitled "Discovery of the Cystic Fibrosis Gene (1989)"[1] Salvador Galdamez writes about the day the gene for CF was finally discovered: Richard Rozmahel had read "yet another variation of the same tedious experiment." But this time something about the printout of results stopped him. He saw something quite different from anything he had seen before. He noticed that "there is a three-base pair deletion . . . a type of genetic mutation in a DNA sequence. The genetic information required to describe one amino acid in a protein chain is missing." Suddenly, the missing piece was right in front of him. His supervisor, Dr. Tsui, senior scientist and Sellers Chair of Cystic Fibrosis Research in the Department of Genetics at the Research Institute of the Hospital for Sick Children in Toronto, was on hand to hear the exciting news.

"I am pretty sure I've found a three-base pair deletion," Rozmahel explained, pointing excitedly to the trace from a healthy person's genes and the trace from a person who has cystic fibrosis. It took another five months of work by Dr. Tsui and his lab personnel to prove that they had in fact found the gene that causes CF. Their hypothesis was confirmed and the results were published in September 1989.

Today, the following is understood about the gene that causes CF, known as the CFTR gene: The CFTR gene is a large gene that codes for many amino acids to make up a protein. CFTR is responsible for balancing the salt content of the cells that line the lungs and certain other organs. "CFTR is supposed to travel to a cell's surface to create openings, or channels, for chloride ions to exit that cell. But cells police protein quality, trapping mutated CFTR and shuttling it to a holding bin for later destruction. Thus, chloride can't escape, and an eventual salt buildup inside cells leads to the dangerous mucus formation."[2]

There are three bases in the gene that codes for each amino acid, and in the case of Delta F508 mutation, there is a deletion of three bases (CTT), which leads to a loss of the protein phenylalanine at position 508. But the same gene can have another mutation at another position. Considering that the CFTR consists of something like 1,500 amino acids, it comes as little surprise that there can be other mutations in the same gene, although it is not very common. The 1,500 amino acids would correspond to 4,500 bases, and only one base flaw is needed to cause a mutation. A person who has CF can have two mutations on the same gene. If this person then has a child who has CF, the child should have the same two mutations on the gene he inherited from the parent.[3]

This might be somewhat difficult and too scientific to follow if you do not have a background in genetics or even in biology. So, all of this basically means that there are quite a large number of mutations—over seven hundred, it is believed—that, when paired, can cause a person to be born with cystic fibrosis.

Whether or not the inherited mutation combination has any bearing on the symptoms he or she experiences remains unclear. However, given the fact that symptoms can vary widely from sibling to sibling within the same family, one would have to surmise that mutations themselves do not account for the severity of the illness. But what does all of this mean in terms of the big questions of *how* and *why*?

ANOTHER BOOK WORTH READING

Blow the House Down: The Story of My Double Lung Transplant **by Charlie Tolchin (Lincoln, NE: Writers Club Press, 2000) is an inspiring chronicle of the author's battle with cystic fibrosis and the double lung transplant that saved his life.**

There remains no cure for cystic fibrosis. But almost every day there is new information coming forth, full of hope and promise, such as drug trials for new and better medicines and therapy devices, the promise of gene therapy, and improved outcomes from lung transplant surgery.

One day there will undoubtedly be a cure for cystic fibrosis. In the meantime, managing CF for each individual who has cystic fibrosis remains the best and only defense. People who have cystic fibrosis are living longer now than ever before. Yet, the reality is that there are still young people who don't make it out of their teens and still others who don't even make it into their teens. Attitude is key but must be coupled with a good daily regimen of treatments and a strong dose of luck.

"I never expected to be around at 30, but I'm 25 now, and I think I'll see the next five years. But beyond that, it's hard to see. I guess I could live to be 35, but that might be a stretch. I can't really predict beyond five years. My CF has progressed in the past five years. I still consider my health to be relatively good. I've outlived most of my friends from CF camp. I think the odds are with me.

"I don't think I'll get married. I would live with someone, though. I think it would be hard for me to be the mate of someone who doesn't have CF. CF is such an everyday thing with so many little nuisances. I think I'd find it difficult to open up that much to someone who did not already understand exactly what I deal with every day. I think it would be easier to be with someone who also has CF."—Chad Lucci

According to the CF Foundation's National Patient Registry, the median age of survival for a person with CF is 35.1 years.[4]

There are some who believe that the "just around the corner" cure is still too elusive. "We've been hearing about the cure coming soon for over ten years now" could be a quote attributed to just about anyone who has CF. So many people have died waiting for that cure. While there is a strong possibility that one day cystic fibrosis will be a disease that takes up space only in history books, whether or not that day will be in our lifetime remains to be seen. Optimistically, some feel certain a cure is very close. Others feel there might only be a continued improvement of maintenance drugs. While the future is uncertain, those who have CF are generally happy to know that research is being conducted on their behalf. They are grateful for the steady stream of new medicines and therapies becoming available on a somewhat regular basis. While none of these provides a cure, they do improve prognosis. And they might help some people who have cystic fibrosis live long enough and stay healthy enough to possibly benefit from a cure. Others might argue that living longer could open them up to the possibility—and probability—of developing more problems related to CF. However, most people who have CF seem to feel that—given the choice—they would rather take a new medication and live with the consequences of aging with cystic fibrosis than not have the opportunity to live at all.

BETTER DRUGS, BETTER PROGNOSIS

New drugs are being tested regularly. According to the Cystic Fibrosis Foundation, in coming years you are likely to start hearing about new medications with names like Compacted DNA, Curcumin, Vertex, Parion, Nacystelyn, Lomucin, and TheraCLEC, all of which are either currently in the initial testing phase in a laboratory or have already progressed to human safety trials. These new drugs are being developed in the hope of improving treatment for nutritional issues, regulating mucus, reducing inflammation, and possibly even effecting a cure as in the case of two drugs being tested as possible gene therapy. People who have CF discuss how well one new medicine is working, while working out the kinks of another. New ideas, new drug trials, and new discoveries come up so frequently that even as this book takes shape, new developments pop up regularly, and inclusion of all of these drugs would be impossible. Not to mention the fact that a list would be both incomplete and outdated by the time you are reading this. Suffice it to say that researchers are working on the problem.

"There are some new Zithromax trials. We have a couple of patients in our CF center who take Zithromax on a regular basis. It has a profound anti-inflammatory action as well as being a pretty good antibiotic. I believe the 'evidence-based jury' is still out though," says Mike Shoemaker, a respiratory therapist in Easley, South Carolina, regarding promising new drugs on the horizon.

Over the last two decades or so, much has changed in the way cystic fibrosis is treated. Because more is understood about the disease itself, different and better treatments have replaced less effective ways of managing CF. Joanne Schum is 40 years old. She had a lung transplant a few years ago, so she is dealing with a new set of challenges. Meanwhile, one question about her life remains constant, "How did you live so long with CF when the prognosis forty years ago was nothing close to today's thirty-three years?" Joanne shares her ideas about what kept her and her sister alive past the "average" as she describes changes in CF care over the years.

Did You Know?
Sandra Boynton, author and illustrator of such children's books as *Pajama Time*, *Barnyard Dance*, and *Philadelphia Chickens*, has donated $21,000 to the CF Foundation through her charitable foundations Echo Valley Foundation and Workman Publishing's Whispering Bells Foundation. With two coworkers' children diagnosed with cystic fibrosis, Boynton decided to dedicate a portion of her book sales to the CF Foundation.[5]

Katherine L. Shores was the oldest living person with CF in the United States. She turned 79 on July 1, 2004! She died on Sunday, November 21, 2004.[6]

"When I was diagnosed at four years old my parents were told to expect me to live to about 10 years old. So why am I here at 40 and my sister at 50? We supposedly have a gene that is not as serious as others. [Note: It is questionable whether or not some mutations or mutation combinations actually produce a more or less severe case of CF. After all, siblings who have CF have the same mutations, yet the course of their illness might be dramatically different, such as the situation with siblings Olivia and Kevin Pence, whom you read about in chapter 3.] Also, we both had lung transplants. I had mine when I was 33, and my sister had hers at 46.

"I've been asked how the world of CF has changed in my lifetime and whether or not TOBI® and Pulmozyme are credited for the longevity of my sister and me. When I was young, we only had a few antibiotics to take. Maybe it was penicillin, in fact. There were no nebulized meds, no inhalers, and I am sure IV antibiotics were not used much. I had my first IV at 14 years old. Clapping, cupping, or chest physiotherapy was the big thing for my sister and me. We started with the old-fashioned clapping by my parents. Then we got some various electric things that would pound us; one looked like a drill, another like a jigsaw. None of them worked great. Neither my sister nor I ever had a Vest. She used a sonic percussor, and I used the old-fashioned hand cupping.

"So, what kept us alive and what was the most beneficial, I believe, was the progress made in the field of CF during our early years. There were new drugs, new therapies, and new IV meds, and we thank our doctor for using these when they became available. My sister and I started Pulmozyme the day it came out. We were so excited. It was the cure for us! I give that a lot of credit for keeping me healthy. I never used TOBI®. It was not yet available. It came out a few months after I got new lungs. The other big benefit, I feel, was prednisone. I know people hate it and the side effects can be nasty, but I truly believe that prednisone allowed me to live longer without needing a lung transplant, and it literally kept me alive. I feel I would be dead had I not been put on it around age 20. I [also] have excellent control of my diabetes, and it has never been a problem for me. Another thing I give credit to is physical activity. As we were growing up, they kept instilling in us to 'stay active, swim, bike, walk, and so forth.' This was not easy for me. I was not athletic, nor did I have any real interest in sports. But I know that when I started to work out at the YMCA, I discovered the many benefits—both mental and physical—of walking on the track. It was a joy! My love for walking began, and I truly know that helped me to sustain my old CF lungs longer. Those are my ideas as to why I'm still around, anyway."—Joanne Schum

"As for the question of where the research dollars are going . . . all of the areas affected by the CFTR protein regulator abnormality are areas where Cystic Fibrosis Foundation research money is being funneled. Many of the new areas of research focus on repairing the broken chloride channel, which leads to the sticky mucus that causes CF symptoms in both the lungs and the gastrointestinal (GI) tract. However, specifically for the GI tract, there is currently a new enzyme and an infant formula in Phase I trial and an observation study on the complications of CF-related diabetes. Also, there is a Phase I trial on the treatment of bone loss (which is related to the malabsorption from GI issues)."—Kirsten M. Black, coordinator of special events, Georgia chapter of the Cystic Fibrosis Foundation

In conclusion, Ms. Black assures us that the CF Foundation is well aware of—and working toward better understanding and treatment of—the issues other than pulmonary involvement.

A CURE?

Perhaps the most promising hope for a cure for cystic fibrosis is gene therapy. Since 1993 at least one hundred people who have cystic fibrosis have undergone treatment with gene therapy. Still in research and test trial phase, gene therapy is administered by inhaling a spray that contains normal copies of the CF gene that have been spliced into vectors. The corrected copy of the CF gene is inhaled and delivered to the lungs. Yet another promising therapy is protein repair therapy. Protein repair therapy would repair the defective CFTR protein.[7] Still, there remains no cure for cystic fibrosis.

Meanwhile, as treatments get better and better, people who have CF are, on average, living longer and longer. This has led to the need for a new type of CF care: adult care.

IN THE MEANTIME: MAKING THE TRANSITION FROM PEDIATRIC HOSPITAL TO ADULT CF CENTER

Not long ago, the need for adult CF centers became apparent. Now no longer a disease confined solely to childhood, young adults and a growing number of older adults began requiring care beyond the scope of their pediatric CF doctors. Adult CF centers began springing up in the major cities, usually pairing themselves with existing pediatric CF centers.

Those making the transition had mixed emotions about leaving their childhood CF centers behind. Many were well into their 20s and even older when the option to go to an adult hospital became available. Many were given the choice to transition or to remain in their pediatric centers. For some people the transition was easy and natural; for others, it was not such a pleasure.

Approximately 40 percent of the CF population is 18 years old or older.

"Why did I decide to make the switch? My doctors asked me to when I was about 15, 17, somewhere in there. I was hesitant because I had grown comfortable with my doctors over the eight years that I had been going to Children's Memorial. But when I was admitted and assigned to a room with a 2-year-old, that's when I decided it was time to go to an adult hospital! I had actually been to an adult hospital when I was away at school in San Diego, and I went to an adult clinic in Iowa while I finished up school there. When I came back to Chicago after graduation, I saw some of the adult clinic doctors at Children's.

Then I moved to Northwestern's adult program when I was about 21 or 22. The transition was nice. The hospital was so nice. It's different because I'm no longer treated like a special kid with an illness as we were at Children's. That was great when I was a kid, but I no longer needed that as an adult. I was ready for the change."—Chad Lucci

"Starting in my mid-20s, I started seeing the pediatric and adult doctor on an alternating basis at Johns Hopkins, so I could get used to them. Finally, the switch was made permanent in 1997 or so. I've been real happy with my adult team. But while I was in my 20s, I was still seeing the pediatric team. Well, I just learned to live with it. After all, I needed them too much."
—Mike L., 30, Baltimore, Maryland

"My daughter Kris transferred to the adult clinic at her hospital, but it was like a combined pediatric and adult situation. She loved the doctor and was very happy. But then the wonderful doctor left, and the replacement should not have been allowed to treat anyone. He had no personality, was rude, and was not capable of treating a person who has CF. He was new to the hospital, and Kris was the first person to transfer to his care. It was terrible. Not only did her health suffer, but she also hated going to see him. We are now back in pediatrics and very happy. We would like to try out other clinics, but we are afraid Kris's health might suffer."—Claudia Dunn, Basking Ridge, New Jersey, mother of Kris, 21

"I switched from a children's hospital to an adult hospital in August 2002, and I actually ended up in the adult hospital for the first time in February 2003. I *hated* it. The care is different. I don't know how to explain it. It's rough transferring to adult care, especially when you already have a good team of doctors, and you get used to the way things are done. The way doctors treat children versus adults is different; they are more warmhearted with the kids than they are with adults."—Kelli B., 22, Englewood, Colorado

Do your research before you decide to make the switch. As Chad pointed out, it's no fun rooming with a crying 2-year-old (and his mother!). On the other hand, it can be difficult to give up your comfort zone and start anew with all new medical personnel late in the game. Ask other young adults who have CF whether or not they can honestly recommend the adult CF center in your area. Make an appointment to meet the doctors and nurses and ask them all your questions. In the end, you will have to make the decision that you feel is best for you, both from a medical standpoint and an emotional standpoint.

IF I COULD DO IT ALL OVER AGAIN

On cool August mornings I feel camp the most. I miss it so much that there's an ache, which I try to ignore as I push forward into another day. My days are full of ordinary activities: taking care of my children, writing, cooking, shopping, and seeing my friends. I have learned the hard way not to take my days for granted because so many wonderful young people would have given just about anything to have lived long enough to share each day with me.

It takes very little for me to conjure up memories of CF camp. Usually, it's little more than a song on the radio, something by Air Supply or Wham!, or that old song, "That's What Friends Are For." And then I am overwhelmed with sadness and nostalgia . . . and gratitude.

When I first attended CF camp, I naively though I was going there to "help the kids with cystic fibrosis." How little I understood about life back then. How little I realized all that *I* needed. During that first week, and in the years to follow, I would find, more often than not, that it was the CF kids and young adults who did the "helping." They helped me realize my own potential and all I could do if I just put my mind to it. They taught me that life is short, but it's also beautiful. It sounds so cliché, but it's true that they showed me that the sky is blue and the grass is green and snow is so lovely as it falls. If I could do it all over again I would. I'd start just the same, as an innocent

211

18-year-old who thought she had something to give. Because the gifts I have been given by those I have known who have CF are by far among the most meaningful gifts I could ever have imagined receiving. The benefits of their friendships have far outweighed the risks, no matter how heartbreaking. They put me where I am today, and for that I can only say, "Thank you."

"When are you going to just walk away?" my friend Cathy Carnevale asked me in 1996, just after our friend Mike DiBiase died of complications following his double lung transplant. 'When is this going to be too much for you to deal with?' she asked.

"I'll walk away when you can walk away with me," I told her.

Would I do it all again if I knew up front just how much pain I would endure as I lost friend after friend to this horrible disease? I don't hesitate when I answer, "Yes." Nothing can ever take away the pain of so much loss. But so many good things have come out of my experiences, not the least of which are my two beautiful, healthy, little boys. And these miracles have shown me once and for all that things happen for a reason, even if sometimes the reason takes a long time to reveal itself. The father of my little boys is a man I met and married when we both worked as pediatric respiratory therapists. Yes, I would do it all again.

ANOTHER BOOK WORTH READING

A truly amazing and comprehensive annotated listing of books about cystic fibrosis, both technical and popular, can be found at the Cystic-L online bookstore: cystic-l.org/html/CFS-Bookstore.htm.

IN THEIR OWN WORDS

As with any serious illness, the life lessons learned by those who have CF and those close to them are great. Many of the teens and adults I interviewed for this book had something unique to say about themselves, their lives, and what it means to live with cystic fibrosis.

One can't help but wonder how those who have cystic fibrosis feel about living with their disease. If they were given the opportunity to choose, would they choose to live a life with CF, or would they choose a life of breathing easy? Can there possibly be anything good about having CF? What do they feel is the worst thing about having CF? What advice would a teen or young adult who has CF wish to share with others who are facing the challenges of CF? Their answers might surprise you.

"As much as it's a pain [to have CF], it's made me much stronger. Little things don't bother me because I've been through so much. Having CF and having had two double lung transplants have helped me make some important decisions regarding smoking and drinking. I know the damage that could be done to me if I were to do those things. I value life. I think this makes me fun to be around. It takes a lot to get me down. I'm usually in a good mood. I've had so much more life

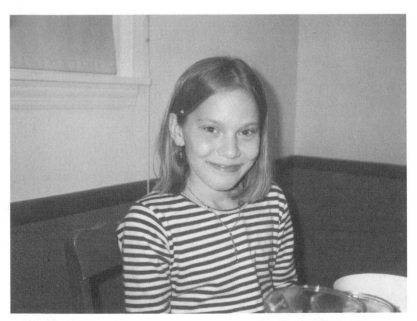

Katie Kocelko was thin and pale and on oxygen most of the time when she turned 11 in June 1996. Shortly after this photo was taken, Katie and her mother went to St. Louis and Katie received her first double lung transplant.

experience than most teenagers. I've learned to just take things in stride, to take bad news easily. When I had my second transplant I was excited, even though I knew what work lay ahead for me. The only thing I was really bummed about was that I had to miss most of my senior year [of high school]. But then I knew this would allow me to go to college. If I could change it all now I would, but maybe not ten years ago because I wouldn't have had so many experiences. I like who I am, who I turned out to be because of my experiences. Yes, from a health point of view, it would be nice to change things, but from a personality point of view, I like things just the way they are."
—Katie Kocelko, 18

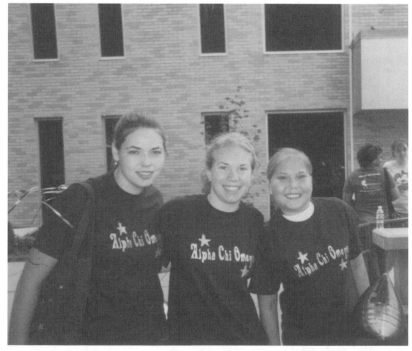

Katie, in 2003, is a healthy, active college student. Pictured here at age 18 with Bradley University sorority sisters, Katie, on the right, still shows signs of puffiness in her face, due to steroids used to keep her body from rejecting her second new pair of lungs.

A CYSTIC FIBROSIS TIMELINE

1936 First clinical description of CF as a distinct disease is made by Swiss physician, Professor Fanconi. Most children born with CF die before their first birthday.

1938 Pathologist Dr. Dorothy Anderson at New York's Columbia University makes first pathological description of cystic fibrosis.

1940s CF is recognized as a generalized disorder and is called "mucoviscidosis." Enzyme supplements are prescribed to help digest food.

1946 Studies of the pattern of cystic fibrosis in families lead researchers to the fact that cystic fibrosis is genetic, a recessive condition, and is most likely caused by a mutation of a single gene.

1949 A Detroit physician and pathologist describes obstruction by abnormal mucus as the principal cause of the progressive lung disease of cystic fibrosis.

1950s Penicillin and other antibiotics are used to fight infection.

1953 Dr. Paul di Sant'Agnese, at National Institutes of Health (NIH) in Bethesda, Maryland, describes salt loss as the reason for the deaths of some dozen or so infants with cystic fibrosis during a heat wave in New York City.

Mid-1950s Cystic fibrosis clinics are up and running in Boston, New York, Baltimore, Philadelphia, and San Francisco.

1955 Cystic Fibrosis Foundation is established to find new treatments for cystic fibrosis and ultimately the cure.

1957 Canada opens its first CF clinic at Montreal Children's Hospital.

1959 Gibson-Cooke pilocarpine iontophoresis procedure for collecting and measuring sweat chloride levels to test children for CF is published, replacing previous crude efforts to measure sweat salt concentrations.

Late 1950s Doctors realize they are doing children a disservice by waiting until they get sick to begin treatment for CF. Methods are changing to initiate treatment as soon as a diagnosis is made in an attempt to prevent lung damage.

1960s Children sleep in mist tents to moisten their lungs.

1966 Nova Scotia, Canada, reports forty-six residents with CF. The oldest is 20 years old, but the majority are younger than 12 years old.

1989 Gene responsible for causing cystic fibrosis is discovered.

1990 Significant progress is made in experiments with a potential new CF treatment: the aerosol administration of Dornase Alpha (DNAse). ThAIRapy Vest aids in chest therapy.

1993 DNAse is approved by the FDA. Doctors begin researching gene therapy as a cure.

1999 Nova Scotia, Canada, reports 175 persons living with CF. The oldest is 38 years old.[8]

It has often been said that with every bad thing there is something good. Of course, the opposite might be true as well. Those who have CF find that, for the most part, there is always something good that comes from their bad situation. Sometimes the things they find are very serious and life affirming and sometimes they might seem trivial, but whatever it is, good is good!

The Best Thing about Having Cystic Fibrosis Is . . .

"The life experience—being more aware of decisions, being in control of my life and cherishing life, knowing how precious it is."—Katie Kocelko

**How can you be strong
When you're frail
How can you believe
When you're hopeless
How can you love life
When you're in Hell
How can you be yourself
When you're overpowered
How can you understand
When you're confused
How can you see
When you're oblivious
How can you live
When you're dying
How can you be like everyone else
When you're different
How can you dream
When you're awake
How can you be beautiful
When you're a mess
How can you have faith
When you're not certain
How can you trust
When you're scared
—Leah K.**

"Probably realizing who your true friends are and who is willing to go through deep waters with you. Having CF also means that you appreciate life more, and you don't take your health for granted."—Alice Vosloo

@

"The people I've met that I most likely wouldn't have if I didn't have CF. Often, if I think back on how I met people, I end up realizing I may well not have met them if it weren't for some circumstance related to CF. Also, it helps keep things in perspective, I think. For example, I seriously doubt I'll be griping about wrinkles and prostate exams and so on when it comes times for those."—James Lawlor

Did You Know?
The agent of New York Jets quarterback Jay Fiedler has a daughter who has CF.

@

"The best thing to me is realizing who I am and what I'm worth. The hard times have kept me grounded and have made my faith in God a lot stronger. I am willing to help others like me, and the desire to do so keeps me going. I don't take things for granted. I consider each morning I wake up as another gift."—Jessica Hawk-Manus

@

"You get to miss school and you never have to diet!"—Krystal Freake

@

"CF has made me the person I am. Without it, I know that I would be a different person. I thank God each day for everything I have and am able to do. I don't take the simple things for granted, and I cherish the simplest accomplishment. CF has made me a stronger person. When I have to do IVs or when I've just had a bad week, I can bounce back. I know that things could be worse, and I take the bad days with a grain of salt. I have been through a lot, both CF related and non-CF related, and will have to go through much more, but with every day I live, my will gets a little stronger."—Jackie Goryl

"I can eat whatever I want. I know it sounds silly but look at how many people are on diets. With CF, you never need one except, maybe, a high-calorie diet with lots of chocolate!" —Janelle Benitez

"I don't think there is one."—Chad Lucci

On the other hand, having a disease like cystic fibrosis can certainly have its downside. In fact, at times it can be downright difficult.

The Worst Thing about Having Cystic Fibrosis Is . . .

"I guess knowing that it will get worse as time goes on, and that if a cure isn't found, CF will probably be what kills you. Of course, not feeling well, being sick, and so on, isn't all that great either, but you get used to it (somewhat) after awhile."—James Lawlor

"The pain and the uncertainty. While knowing that each day could be your last makes you strong, it also makes you weak at the same time. It's scary."—Jessica Hawk-Manus

"The worst thing about having CF is thinking about it. Having to do treatments every day. If I stay out late, I still have to do my treatment when I get home, even if I'm too tired. And if I skip the treatment, I know I'll get sick. It's just always in my face."—Maggie Sheehan

"Not being able to go on camping trips or sleepovers (because I won't get any sleep), having to cough all the time, especially in

a movie or in class, and people always asking if I'm sick."
—Alice Vosloo

◎

"The worst thing is hard to say. I can't decide. It's a toss up among getting sick at the worst times and not being able to do things because of it, doing therapy twice a day, or watching your friends die. I guess, overall, it's watching your friends die. As far as personally, it would be getting sick at the most inopportune times."
—Janelle Benitez

◎

"Looking young."—Katie Kocelko

◎

Did You Know?
Jerry McMorris, owner of the Colorado Rockies, had a son named Mike who had CF.[9]

"Living my whole life knowing I am going to pass before everyone my age. Knowing my friends will grow up, marry, and have kids and I won't."—Chad Lucci

◎

"Constantly coughing and also being prevented from playing sports when I'm sick."—Krystal Freake

◎

"The uncertainty of not knowing my future. I won't lie. There are times when I wonder if college, boyfriends, and so forth, are worth it. Will I find someone and only have a year or two with him? With this disease, you just don't know. Treating adults is like uncharted territory. Doctors are unfamiliar with the effects of CF on the adult body, so they are learning as we grow. It is hard to not be able to control what happens. To do everything you are supposed to and know that it might not make you any better is frustrating."—Jackie Goryl

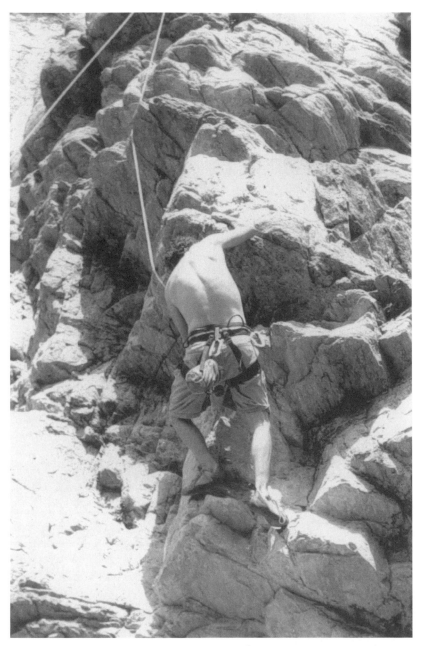

Chad Lucci partaking in one of his favorite activities, rock/mountain climbing.

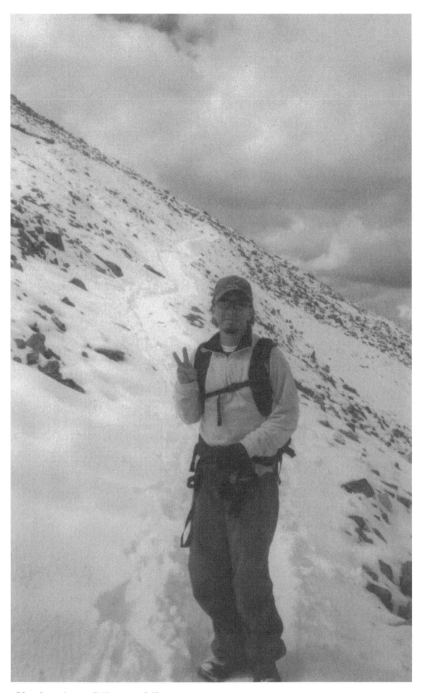

Chad on top of the world!

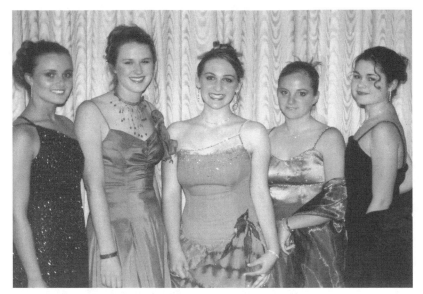

Alice Vosloo, far right, and her friends going to a dance

My Advice to Teens Is . . .

"Hang in there, eventually they'll find a cure, but 'till then, look after yourself, 'cause they won't be able to reverse damage done."—Alice Vosloo, 19

"Try to get the most out of friendships and family while you're healthy. Experience the most out of life. I don't mean doing drugs and drinking; I mean the good, healthy experiences life has to offer."—Chad Lucci, 25

"Live every day to the fullest and don't take anything for granted. CF is a tough disease, but things could still be worse. There is a reason you have CF; God knew you could handle it. Think about the things you have done and the things you will do, and know that CF will not hinder your successes; it will only make you push harder to fulfill those dreams. I like to think that I have proved everyone wrong. When I was diagnosed, they said I wouldn't graduate high school or go to college. In June 2004 I will graduate from college. Don't think about the things you cannot do, but think about the things you have done. Thank those around you for the support and love they have shown you. Don't be afraid or embarrassed of your CF because that will only hold you back. CF has made me a stronger person, and it has done something for you too. And finally, do what every other person your age is doing: dream, hope, and love."—Jackie Goryl, 23

⊚

"Don't lose faith or hope. *Never* lose either of these. Both of these qualities make you so much stronger, more so than you could ever realize. Always believe in yourself."—April Harris-Kinsey, 20

⊚

"Try to always look at the positive side even if things are hard. Take the life experiences, and see how much more mature it makes you. And also, try to make friends with other teens who have CF."—Katie Kocelko, 18

⊚

"Hang in there. Being a teenager is tough, even without a chronic illness. I remember feeling sorry for myself many times as a teenager, blaming CF for most of it. I know that there are times when the treatments and the medications seem pointless, and you just want to quit everything all together. But as you get older, it does get easier. You will come across people who are more mature and understanding. There's nothing to be ashamed of because this is who you are. You've got a lot of things to do in your future, so take care of yourself so that you can be as healthy as possible for it."—Leah K., 23

⊚

"Keep a positive attitude, take CF seriously, and do everything possible to keep healthy, and enjoy life while we're here to do so."—James Lawlor, 17

⊚

"Don't let CF define who you are. Stay strong and stay tough. There is hope out there for us. Attitude affects our health more than the disease itself does. Strong people with good attitudes can make it through *anything*. Pray, and do it often."—Jessica Hawk-Manus, 25

⊚

"I would say hang in there, it gets better and easier. Also, enjoy yourself; try to do as many normal teen things as possible from toilet papering your school to going to dances or whatever you and your friends like to do. Don't hold back because of CF; try things. Something I wish someone had told me: exercise, you won't regret it. Find a sport or activity you like and do it. For motivation, do some vigorous activity instead of therapy. [But talk to your CF doctor first.] Swimming, running, or biking always makes me cough more than any therapy. If people tease you or make jokes about you because you're sick or miss school a lot, then they are not worth knowing. Try not to let it bother you, teenagers are cruel, that's why I say hang in there, it gets better."
—Janelle Benitez, 25

"There are always people who are worse off than you."
—Krystal Freake, 16

ANOTHER ADULT DECISION: COLLEGE

My parents had driven me back to school to begin my sophomore year of college. The RA (resident advisor, the student in charge of all the students living on her dorm floor) made her rounds, introducing herself to each of the new students on her floor. She was a senior and her name was Karen. It was unusual for me to meet a girl who was shorter than my own petite stature of five feet tall. I listened to her talk and took note of other subtleties of her appearance. When she departed and was surely out of earshot, I said to my mom, "Karen has CF."

"No she doesn't," my mom replied. "You just got back from CF camp. You just have CF on your mind."

"Right," I said, "I do have CF on my mind because I just spent a week with kids who have CF, and I know what I am looking at!" My mother still thought I was seeing something that was not there, so she suggested I mention my involvement with CF camp to Karen. Eventually I did but to no avail. I had to tell my mom that perhaps she was right, though I still believed Karen had CF. It wasn't until later, in September, that I was stumbling down the dorm hall, blinded by tears and pain having just learned that my friend Angela Dibbern had died, that Karen caught me and *pulled me into her room. Perhaps to console and reassure me, or perhaps to offer some understanding, Karen finally admitted, "I have CF." My reply was a simple, tearful, "I know."*

That was 1987. I don't know what has become of Karen, although I do know that she earned her degree and graduated that year. What I found most impressive about Karen was that she had made it. She had CF, she was away at school, in charge of a floor of sometimes rowdy and emotional teenage girls, she took care of her own medical needs, without access to the modern conveniences of the Vest or the Flutter, and she was graduating. Her family had probably been told that she wouldn't live past her fifth birthday.

The question of whether or not to attend college has only been a real issue for a relatively short number of years. When the median age of survival for someone with CF was only fifteen years, whether or not to attend college never even made it to discussion. But today, with improved prognosis, more and more young people who have cystic fibrosis are planning for their own futures alongside their healthy peers. However, unlike their healthy peers, some minor (and not so minor) accommodations need to be planned for more carefully. Janice Poling, 25, of Hyattsville, Maryland, double majored in geological sciences and history at Case Western Reserve University in Cleveland, Ohio, then went on to earn a master's degree from Boston University. Janice makes the following suggestions for a smooth four years of college. "While I was in college, I did the following, and I recommend that others with CF do the same."

◎ **Register with the university's disabilities coordinator. One time I went into the hospital on short notice and the disabilities coordinator called all my professors and explained my situation to them, cut through some red tape to get extensions on some things, and managed to get a laptop for me to use in the hospital in less than an hour (after numerous people told us that borrowing a laptop from the university would be impossible).**

⌾ Tell each of your professors at the beginning of the semester that you have CF and what that means for attending class, such as coughing (for example, explaining that you are not contagious, you cough all the time, and not to worry about you), and that sometimes you end up in the hospital and on IVs. Giving a heads up at the beginning of the semester gave me more credibility if I needed accommodations made later on. Additionally, I always tried to ask for extensions, and so forth, before things were due, so that my professors would know why I was asking, and I might even try to produce evidence that I was really sick (though sometimes this was hard or unnecessary).

In addition, you ought to consider the following points:

⌾ Check to be sure the city in which your university is located has a reputable CF center. You may need it if you get sick or run low on medications.

⌾ Consider choosing a school far enough from home so that you are able to truly enjoy the college experience and are not popping in on your parents every weekend, yet close enough to home that in an emergency you can get home (or your family can get to you with little fuss). Three to six hours away by car seems like a reasonable distance.

⌾ Request a room in a dorm that has air conditioning for those months when it's still warm out.

⌾ Request a single room, which you should be able to get for the price of a double room, as this is a medical necessity. Admittedly, this accommodation could have certain social drawbacks that you'll have to weigh against the privacy advantages. On the other hand, Janice adds, "I had no trouble still being very social. In fact, my room was a pretty popular place to be when it was hot outside because I had the room with the AC!"

⌾ If a single room is unavailable, be sure to request a roommate who does not smoke.

Many people say that their college years are the best years of their lives. Take care of yourself, don't neglect your health, and enjoy your four years away. There is nothing else like being away at college!

IS THAT IT, THEN?

In a nutshell, no. There is much to be learned about cystic fibrosis, both from a social point of view and a medical perspective. Even as this book comes to its conclusion, there is no closure on the topic of cystic fibrosis. Not yet, anyway. Clinical trials for various medications are ongoing, discoveries continue to be made, and new questions provoke new answers, which in turn provoke further questions. Mothers are learning that they are carrying fetuses who will be born with CF. Babies are still being born with cystic fibrosis every day. Children and teens are enduring daily rounds of therapy and frequent hospitalizations in an effort to slow the path of this life-threatening disease. Adults are learning to live with a disease that was once considered a childhood disease. And, worst of all, children, teens, and adults still die of cystic fibrosis every day.

It all comes down to the desperate need for a cure. Until there is a cure for cystic fibrosis, the story of what it's like to live with this disease is an ongoing one, with no real ending—not yet.

I've spent more than half my life now involved with cystic fibrosis. Not because I had to but because I chose to. I have said good-bye to more friends than I care to count (although I have counted, and the number is a staggering fifty-six). Like those who have cystic fibrosis and those who care for them every day, I too look forward to the day when, in the words of 8-year-old Alex Deford, "they find a cure for my disease, and we all dress up and have a big party." And what a grand party that will be.

NOTES

1. Salvador Galdamez, "Discovery of the Cystic Fibrosis Gene," 1989, www.quasar.ualberta.ca/edse456/apt/vignettes/cystic.htm.
2. Laura Neergaard, "Spice Substance May Fight Cystic Fibrosis," Associated Press, Washington, D.C., April 22, 2004.
3. Johanna Snellman, jsnellman@bton.ac.uk.
4. Cystic Fibrosis Foundation, cff.org/about_cf/what_is_cf.cfm? CFID=1619012&CFTOKEN=84991526.

5. Cystic Fibrosis Foundation.

6. Norma Kennedy Plourde's Cystic Fibrosis website, personal.nbnet.nb.ca/nnormap/CF.htm or www3.nbnet.nb.ca/normap/cfhistory.htm.

7. Kids Health for Parents, websrv02.kidshealth.org/parent/medical/digestive/cf.html.

8. Norma Kennedy Plourde's Cystic Fibrosis website; Ben Whitford, "An Unexpected Reprieve," *Newsweek*, September 12, 2005.

9. Norma Kennedy Plourde's Cystic Fibrosis website.

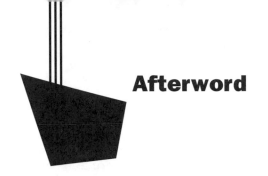

Afterword

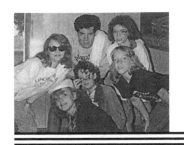

Jessica Hawk-Manus received her double lung transplant in January 2004.

April Harris-Kinsey was married on March 13, 2004. She received a double lung transplant in the summer of 2004. She died in late 2005 while awaiting a kidney transplant.

Leah K. graduated from college in April 2004, earning her bachelor's degree in nursing. She is engaged to be married.

Mike Maggio, associate artistic director of Chicago's Goodman Theatre since 1987, died of complications from post-transplant lymphoma in August 2000 at age 49, nine years post transplant.

Krystal Freake was granted a Make-A-Wish in 2004 and got to travel to Hawaii with her family.

Candice Budnieski graduated in the spring of 2004 with honors from Illinois State University with a Bachelor of Science in Biology. She is enrolled in a two-year Physician's Assistant Program at Finch University. She hopes to make a difference in the health care field. She has suffered a bout with liver pain, frighteningly reminiscent of the complication that took her sister Angela's life in October 2003.

April Budnieski has decided to practice either medical malpractice or family law since her sister Angela's death and will graduate from law school in 2005.

Katie Kocelko completed her freshman year at Bradley University and began her sophomore year in August 2004.

Chad Lucci returned to Chicago to live near his family in the spring of 2004. He is pursuing a degree to become a physician's assistant.

Afterward

Maggie Sheehan turned 16 in March 2004 and got her driver's license.

Maggie Sheehan's friend Devon died in the winter of 2004 at the age of 15.

Jeremy Becker received his double lung transplant on February 15, 2005, after just over a year on the waiting list. Jeremy's posttransplant lung functions were terrific and he thoroughly enjoyed life with new lungs. Unbeknownst to anyone, Jeremy's body harbored a dormant infection prior to transplant, which, once his immune system was suppressed, began to run rampant through his system. Jeremy died of massive infection on Father's Day, June 19, 2005. He was 23 years old.

And the rest continue their valiant fight to beat cystic fibrosis every day.

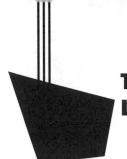

The Fabulous
List of CF Resources

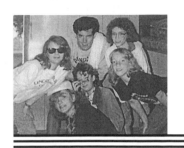

Access to the Internet provides for an ever-changing and growing set of resources. The following websites were found to be helpful to those seeking information about cystic fibrosis in 2003 and 2004. Some websites may have been moved, changed, or removed from the Internet. Others have been added. This list should serve as a springboard for your own research.

WEBSITES

Abe Books, www.abebooks.com. Specializes in older, hard-to-find, and out-of-print books and is a good source for purchasing many of the early books about CF.

Camp Mosquito, www.campmosquito.freeservers.com. Camp Mosquito Lung Disease Adventure Camp.

Canadian Cystic Fibrosis Foundation (CCFF), www.cysticfibrosis.ca. Their official website has copies of excellent CCFF publications about CF, research updates, lists of CF treatments, clinics, and centers, and so forth.

Cell Science, cellscience.com/CFMedical.html. List of international CF centers.

CF Pharmacy, www.cfpharmacy.com. CF Pharmacy is "dedicated to research and development of a new cost-effective pharmaceutical approach to the care and treatment of cystic fibrosis. The CF Pharmacy is an independent pharmacy for patients and families across the United States formed specifically to meet the needs of CF patients. In addition to medication, the CF Pharmacy carries a full line of respiratory equipment and supplies as well as nutritional supplements."

CF Roundtable, www.cfroundtable.com. A newsletter for adults who have CF.

Clear Lake Pros, www.clearlakepros.com/campfunshine/ home_sm.html. Camp Funshine, CF camp.

Compassionate Friends, www.compassionatefriends.org. Compassionate Friends is a national group with local chapters specifically for people who experience the death of a child (of any age).

CysticFibrosis.com, cysticfibrosis.com/kids/stories.htm. Support and information for teachers whose students have CF.

Cystic Fibrosis Foundation, www.cff.org. Resource of CF information.

Cystic Fibrosis Research, Inc. (CFRI), www.cfri.org/indexframes.htm. "Mission is to fund cystic fibrosis research and to offer educational and support programs for people with CF and their families."

Cystic Fibrosis Worldwide, www.cfww.org. Promotes access to appropriate care and education to people living with CF in developing countries and to improve the knowledge of CF among medical professionals and governments worldwide.

Cystic-L, www.Cystic-L.com. *The* website to visit in your search for understanding what it's like to live with CF. Includes a Links section and a list serve of hundreds of extraordinary people who have CF and parents/grandparents of kids who have CF. This is the *ultimate* CF resource.

Dream Foundation, www.dreamfoundation.com/index.html. The first national organization granting dreams to terminally ill adults (eighteen and older).

Ethan M. Roberts Foundation, www.fightforethan.com. Fighting for the awareness of cystic fibrosis.

Excite directory, www.excite.co.uk/directory/Health/ Conditions_and_Diseases/Genetic_Disorders/Cystic _fibrosis/Camps. Lists CF camps in the United States.

Make-A-Wish Foundation, www.wish.org. This foundation "grants the wishes of children with life-threatening medical conditions."

Milan Foundation, www.facesofcf.com. "This is a place where you can create your own page(s) and tell your story," according to the site's director, Lisa Tucker, mother of a 6-year-old girl with CF.

——— , www.milanfoundation.org. Help for families managing day-to-day needs of people with CF.

MSN Groups, groups.msn.com/TransplantSupport LungHeartLungHeart. Pre- and post-transplant information and support.

National Children's Foundation, www.believeintomorrow.org. The Dreamsurfer Central website is open to children and teenagers ages 8 to 18 who suffer from life-threatening illnesses. Includes moderated chats, games, discussions, message boards, and a site library.

Plourde, Norma Kennedy, www3.nbnet.nb.ca/normap/CF.htm. Impressively well researched, Norma Kennedy Plourde's comprehensive website of all things related to CF is the place to go for more in-depth and up-to-date information.

Protocol Driven Healthcare, Inc., www.mycysticfibrosis.com. Free resource for people living with CF. Tools and resources enabling site members (physicians, patients, caregivers) to "exchange important information to help ensure optimal living with cystic fibrosis."

Reach for the Stars Foundation, www.r4stars.org. This foundation "is dedicated to providing individuals afflicted with cystic fibrosis and their families with the resources, knowledge, and support necessary to manage their unrelenting battle with this insidious disease. We are devoted to improving the quality of life for these afflicted individuals as they await the cure, and to help ease the burden of the families as they engage in their battle with CF."

Second Wind Lung Transplant Association, 2ndwind.org. Everything you ever wanted to know about lung transplants is found in the Second Wind Lung Transplant handbook.

Shark, Irri, www.hometown.aol.com/irrishark/page/index.htm. Shark's personal site including research, links, memorials, and a photo of a Mic-Key g-tube.

Stoddard, Gilbert, www.gilbertstoddard.ca. Gilbert Stoddard's "whole double lung transplant adventure, including dry runs, and lots of transplant pictures."

Through the Looking Glass, www.thebreathingroom.org/lg/lg_mc01_accept. Images of adults with CF.

Yahoo Groups, health.groups.yahoo.com/groups/KidsTouchedByCF. Kids-only site for children with cystic fibrosis and their siblings.

BOOKS

Blau, Eric. *Common Heroes: Facing a Life-Threatening Illness.* Troutdale, OR: NewSage Press, 1989.

Bluebond-Langner, Myra, Bryan Lask, and Denise B. Angst, eds. *Psychosocial Aspects of Cystic Fibrosis.* New York: Oxford University Press, 2001.

Broehl, Dana. *Bittersweet Chances.* Frederick, MD: PublishAmerica, 2004.

Chumbley, Jane. *Cystic Fibrosis: A Family Affair.* London: SPCK and Triangle, 1999.

Deford, Frank. *Alex: The Life of a Child.* Nashville, TN: Rutledge Hill Press, 1997.

Detrich, Terry, and Don Detrich. *The Spirit of Lo: An Ordinary Family's Extraordinary Journey.* Tulsa, OK: Mind Matters, 2000.

Doershuk, Carl F. *Cystic Fibrosis in the 20th Century: People, Events, and Progress.* Guilford, UK: AM Publishing, Ltd., 2002.

Gordon, Jacquie. *Give Me One Wish.* New York: W. W. Norton & Co. Inc., 1988.

Gray, Susan Heinrichs. *Living with Cystic Fibrosis.* Chanhassen, MN: Child's World, 2002.

Harris, Ann, and Maurice Super. *Cystic Fibrosis.* New York: Oxford University Press, 1993.

Hopkins, Karen. *Understanding Cystic Fibrosis*. Understanding Health and Sickness Series. Jackson, MS: University Press of Mississippi, 1998.

Kepron, Wayne. *Cystic Fibrosis: Everything You Need to Know*. Your Personal Health. Willowdale, Canada: Firefly Books, 2004.

Lee, Justin. *Everything You Need to Know About Cystic Fibrosis*. New York: Rosen Publishing, 2001.

Lipman, Andy. *Alive at 25: How I'm Beating Cystic Fibrosis*. Atlanta, GA: Longstreet Press, 2002.

Miller, Robyn. *Robyn's Book: A True Story*. New York: Scholastic, 1986.

Monroe, Judy. *Cystic Fibrosis*. Mankato, MN: Lifematters Press, 2001.

Orenstein, David M. *Cystic Fibrosis: A Guide for Patient and Family*. Hagerstown, MD: Lippincott Williams & Wilkins Publishers, 2003.

Rothberg, Laura. *Breathing for a Living: A Memoir*. New York: Hyperion Press, 2003.

Schum, Joanne M., ed. *Taking Flight: Inspirational Stories in Lung Transplantation*. Victoria, Canada: Trafford, 2002.

Schwartz, Tina P. *How to Survive Your Parent's Organ Transplant: The Ultimate Teen Guide*. Lanham, MD: Scarecrow, 2005.

Widerman, Eileen, Barbara Palys, and John R. Palys, eds. *Now That I Have CF: Information for Men and Women Diagnosed as Adults*. Solvay Pharmaceuticals, 2004.

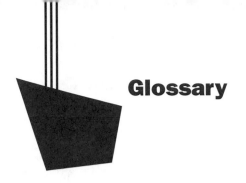

Glossary

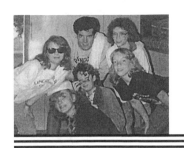

anesthesia The absence of normal sensation, especially to pain, as induced by an anesthetic substance for medical or surgical purposes.

antibiotic Medicine with the ability to destroy or interfere with the development of a living organism.

asthma Respiratory disorder characterized by recurring episodes of paroxysmal dyspnea (episodic shortness of breath), wheezing on expiration/inspiration caused by constriction of the bronchi, coughing, and viscous mucoid bronchial secretions.

autosomal recessive Pattern of inheritance in which the transmission of a recessive gene on an autosome (an ordinary, paired, non–sex chromosome that is the same in both sexes of a species; humans have twenty-two pairs of autosomes) results in a carrier state if the person is heterozygous (carrying two different versions of a gene on the two corresponding chromosomes) for the trait (Aa) and will show the trait if homozygous (carrying two identical copies of a gene on two corresponding chromosomes) (aa) for it.

biliary cirrhosis Inflammatory condition in which the flow of bile through the ductules of the liver is obstructed.

bolus Relatively large amount of intravenous medication or feeding formula administered rapidly to decrease the response time.

CAT scan (also known as CT scan) Computerized Tomography. Radiographic technique that produces film that represents a detailed cross-section of tissue structure.

237

CFTR Cystic Fibrosis Transmembrane Conductance Regulator. Large gene that codes for many amino acids to make up a protein and is responsible for balancing the salt content of the cells that line the lungs and certain other organs. When defective, it causes cystic fibrosis.

colonize Process by which microorganisms multiply without invasion or damage of tissues.

Delta F508 Gene mutation that accounts for approximately 90 percent of all cases of cystic fibrosis.

DNA Deoxyribonucleic acid. Large, double-stranded, helical, nucleic acid molecule found principally in the chromosomes of the nucleus of a cell, which is the carrier of genetic information.

endoscopy Visualization of the interior organs and cavities of the body with an endosope.

ENT Ear, nose, and throat doctor.

enzyme Complex produced by living cells that catalyze chemical reactions in organic matter.

epithelial cells Cells arranged in one or more layers that form part of a covering or lining of a body surface.

genetic Pertaining to reproduction, birth, or origin; produced by a gene; inherited.

GERD Gastroesophageal reflux disease. Backflow of contents of the stomach into the esophagus that is often the result of incompetence of the lower esophageal sphincter. The acidity of the gastric juices produces a burning sensation in the esophagus.

g-tube/gastrostomy tube Tube leading from a surgical creation of an artificial opening into the stomach through the abdominal wall for the purpose of feeding and providing some medications.

hemoptysis Coughing up blood from the respiratory tract.

huff Forced expiration through an open glottis to assist in bringing up mucus before coughing.

insufficiency Inability to perform a necessary function adequately.

in utero Inside the uterus.

IV Intravenous. Giving medicine though a vein.

malabsorption Impaired ability to absorb nutrients from the gastrointestinal tract.

MDI Metered Dose Inhaler. Device designed to deliver a measured dose of an inhaled drug; consists of a canister of aerosol spray, mist, or fine powder that releases a specific dose each time it is pushed against a dispensing valve.

meconium ileus Obstruction of the small intestine in the newborn caused by impaction of thin, dry, tenacious meconium.

MRI Magnetic Resonance Imaging. Spectra emitted by phosphorus in body tissues as measured and imaged on phosphorus, nuclear, magnetic, resonance instruments.

nebulizer Device for producing a fine mist for inhalation.

NG-tube Nasogastric tube. Feeding tube passed into the stomach through the nose.

PICC Line Peripherally Inserted Central Catheter. Long, soft, flexible tube, or catheter, that is inserted through a vein in the arm to reach one of the larger veins located near the heart. It is used to deliver antibiotics, similarly to an IV, but does not need to be changed as often.

pilocarpine Chemical known to enhance sweating, used in the sweat test.

polyp Small, tumorlike growth that projects from the mucous membrane surface.

Pseudomonas aeruginosa Species of gram-negative, non-spore-forming, motile (moving) bacteria that may cause various human diseases.

pulmonary Pertaining to the lungs or the respiratory system.

ROBI Regional Organ Bank of Illinois.

sats Oxygen saturation. The percentage of oxygen in the blood.

Staph A/Staph aureus Species of *Staphylococcus* responsible for certain infections such as boils and abscesses.

Tai Kwon Do A martial art.

toxoplasmosis Common infection with the protozoan intracellular parasite *Toxoplasma gondii*, characterized by rash, lymphadenopathy (an increase in the size of lymph follicles of the lymph nodes, which filter out bacteria and

239

other organisms from the bloodstream), fever, malaise, central nervous system disorders, myocarditis (inflammation of the muscular part of the heart, called the myocardium), and pneumonitis (inflammation of the lung tissue).

tuberculosis Chronic infection by acid-fast bacillus *Myocardium tuberculosis*, transmitted by inhalation or ingestion of infected droplets and usually affecting the lungs.

vas deferens Vessel that conveys sperm.

voracious Greedy, eager eating.

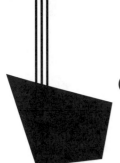

Glossary of CF Meds

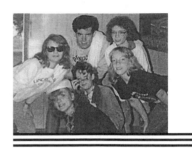

The following are general definitions of the various medications used in treating cystic fibrosis as mentioned in this book.

ADEKS Multivitamin.

Advair An inhalation powder; bronchodilator.

Albuterol A commonly used bronchodilator.

Cipro/Ciprofloxacin An antibiotic.

Colistin An inhaled antibiotic.

Cyclosporine An antirejection drug.

Dilantin An antiseizure drug.

DNAse/Dornase (also known as Pulmozyme) An inhaled expectorant/mucolytic shown to reduce the number of lung infections.

Erythromycin An antibiotic.

Flucoxacillin A penicillin drug that replaced Methicillin.

Gentamycin An antibiotic.

Levaquin (also known as Levofloxacin and Quixin) Broad-spectrum antibiotic.

Methicillin Antibiotic used in the early 1960s to treat *Staph A.*

Mucomyst (also known as acetylcystine and Mucosol) An inhaled medication that lowers viscosity and facilitates removal of secretions.

Pancrease (also known as Pancrelipase) A digestive enzyme.

the Pill Oral birth control.

Prednisone A steroid.

Prevacid (also known as Lansoprazole) Suppresses gastric acid formation in the stomach.

Proventil See Albuterol.

Pulmozyme See DNAse.

Quinolones A class of antibiotics.

Serevent MDI (also known as Salmetrol Xinafoate) An inhaled bronchodilator.

Sporonox (also known as Itraconazole) An antifungal.

TOBI® An inhaled form of the antibiotic Tobramycin.

Tobra/Tobramycin An antibiotic.

Ultrase A digestive enzyme.

Ventolin See Albuterol.

Viokase A digestive enzyme.

Zantac An antiulcer drug.

Zithromax (also known as Azithromycin) An antibiotic.

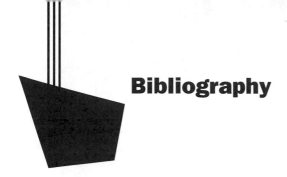

Bibliography

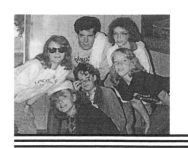

INTERVIEWS WITH AUTHOR

Abrams, Wendy. Questionnaire. Miami: e-mail, 2004.

Anonymous. Questionnaire. Buffalo Grove, IL: e-mail, 2004.

Anonymous. Questionnaire. Chicago: e-mail, 2004.

Apel, Mindy. Short questionnaire. Chicago: e-mail, 2004.

Appel, Michele. Short questionnaire. Elgin, IL: e-mail, 2004.

B., Kelli. Questionnaire. Englewood, CO: e-mail, 2004.

Becker, Jeremy. Questionnaire. Beacon Falls, CT: e-mail, 2004.

Benitez, Janelle. Questionnaire. Michigan: e-mail, 2003.

Black, Kirsten M., coordinator of special events, Cystic Fibrosis Foundation, Georgia chapter. Questionnaire. Atlanta: e-mail, 2004.

Budnieski, Marge. Telephone interview. Mokena, IL, 2004.

———. Questionnaire. Mokena, IL: e-mail, 2004.

Carlson, Rhonda. Short questionnaire. Chicago: e-mail, 2004.

Carnevale, Cathy. Questionnaire. Bolingbrook, IL: e-mail, 2004.

Cherry, Jennifer. Personal interview. Chicago, 1995.

Dexter, Marie. Questionnaire. Kissimmee, FL: e-mail, 2004.

DiBiase, Ken. Personal interview. Chicago, 1995.

DiBiase, Mike. Personal interview. West Chicago, 1996.

Dunn, Claudia. Questionnaire. Basking Ridge, NJ: e-mail, 2004.

Ehrhardt, Tom. Short questionnaire. Glenview, IL: e-mail, 2004.

Fegan-Ehrhardt, Shonne. Short questionnaire. Glenview, IL: e-mail, 2004.

Feinstein, Sam. Questionnaire. Bridgeton, NJ: email, 2004.

Freake, Krystal. Questionnaire. Petit Rocher, New Brunswick, Canada: e-mail, 2003.

French, Kathy. Short questionnaire. Arkansas: e-mail, 2004.

Gibson, Jennie. Questionnaire. Redmond, WA: e-mail, 2004.

Giles, Jo-Anne. Questionnaire. Western Australia: e-mail, 2004.

Gleisten, Samantha. Short questionnaire. Chicago: e-mail, 2004.

Goryl, Jackie. Questionnaire. Kalamazoo, MI: e-mail, 2003.

Hardy, David. Short questionnaire. Modesto, CA: e-mail, 2004.

Harris-Kinsey, April. Questionnaire. Englewood, FL e-mail, 2004.

Hawk-Manus, Jessica. Questionnaire. Nashville, TN: e-mail, 2003.

Jansen, Molly. Questionnaire. Huntersville, NC: e-mail, 2004.

K., Leah. Written questionnaire. Orion, MI: letter, 2003.

Keator, Anne. Questionnaire. Rochester, NY: e-mail, 2003.

Khawaja, Lana. Short questionnaire. Houston: e-mail, 2004.

Kick, Melissa. Telephone interview. Libertyville, IL, 2004.

Kirschbaum, Heidi. Questionnaire. Florida: e-mail, 2004.

Kocelko, Katie. Personal interview. Palatine, IL, 1995.

———. Personal interview. Glenview, IL, 2003.

———. Personal interview. Chicago, 2004.

———. Questionnaire. Peoria, IL: e-mail, 2004.

L., Mike. Questionnaire. Baltimore: e-mail, 2003.

Lawlor, James. Questionnaire. Guntersville, AL: e-mail, 2003.

Lucci, Chad. Telephone interview. Boulder, CO: 2004.

Lucci, Craig. Telephone interview. Evanston, IL, 2003.

McGinty, Alice. Short questionnaire. Urbana, IL: e-mail, 2004.

Meyer, Diane, respiratory therapist, Children's Memorial Hospital. Personal interview. Chicago, 1996.

Monaco, Marcia. Questionnaire. Columbus, OH: e-mail, 2004.

Morey, Brenda. Questionnaire. Placentia, CA: email, 2004.

Mueller, Rebecca. Questionnaire. Philadelphia: e-mail, 2004.

Ottenfeld, Michele. Short questionnaire. Palatine, IL: e-mail, 2004.

Pence, Deborah. Questionnaire. Frankfort, IL: e-mail, 2004.

Pence, Olivia. Questionnaire. Frankfort, IL: e-mail, 2003.

Phillips, Val. Questionnaire. Naples, TX: e-mail, 2004.

Pilarczyk, Kimberlee. Personal interview. Clarendon Hills, IL, 1995.

Poling, Janice. Questionnaire. Hyattsville, MD: email, 2004.

Polski, Donna. Questionnaire. Minnesota: e-mail, 2004.

Pontious, Dawn. Questionnaire. Lexington, SC: e-mail, 2003.

Posteau-Gordon, Stephanie. Short questionnaire. Glenview, IL: e-mail, 2004.

Rodecap, Christine. Questionnaire. Fort Wayne, IN: e-mail, 2003.

Russell, Kathy. Questionnaire. Gresham, OR: email, 2004.

Salazar, Joanne. Children's Memorial Hospital's PFT Lab. Chicago: e-mail, 2004.

Schaab, Meredith. Short questionnaire. Vancouver, British Columbia, Canada: e-mail, 2004.

Schum, Joanne. Questionnaire. New York: e-mail, 2004.

Sheehan, Kerry. Personal interview. Clarendon Hills, IL, 1995.

——. Personal interview. Chicago, 2003.

——. Questionnaire. Chicago: e-mail, 2004.

Sheehan, Maggie. Personal interview. Clarendon Hills, IL, 1995.

——. Personal interview. Clarendon Hills, IL, 2003.

——. Questionnaire. Chicago: e-mail, 2004.

Shoemaker, Mike, respiratory therapist. Questionnaire. Easley, SC: e-mail, 2004.

Smyth, Faela. Questionnaire. Dublin, Ireland: e-mail, 2004.

Snellman, Johanna. Questionnaire. United Kingdom: e-mail, 2004.

Soloff, Harold A., associate, University of London, retired attorney-at-law. Questionnaire. Norwich, CT: e-mail, 2004.

Steading, Cara. Essay. San Antonio, TX, September 2004.

Stoddard, Gil. Questionnaire. Toronto: e-mail, 2004.

Sullivan, Mary. Questionnaire. San Antonio, TX: e-mail, 2004.

Thom, Amy. Personal interview. Joliet, IL: e-mail, 1995.

Thom, Margaret. Personal interview. Joliet, IL, 1995.

Thompson, Sherry. Questionnaire. New York: e-mail, 2004.

———. Questionnaire. New York: letter, 2004.

Tillman, Laura. Questionnaire. Northville, MI: e-mail, 2004.

Villarreal, Veronica. Short questionnaire. Northbrook, IL: e-mail, 2004.

Vosloo, Alice. Questionnaire. Port Elizabeth, South Africa: e-mail, 2003.

White, Melody. Telephone interview. Chicago, January 2006.

Williams, Daelynn. Questionnaire. New London, TX: e-mail, 2004.

X., Henry. Questionnaire. Kansas: e-mail, 2004.

BOOKS

Anderson, Kenneth N., and Lois E. Anderson. *Mosby's Pocket Dictionary of Medicine, Nursing, and Allied Health*. St. Louis: Mosby, 1998.

Deford, Frank. *Alex: The Life of a Child*. Nashville, TN: Rutledge Hill Press, 1997.

Hoff, Patricia Beck, Donald Eitzman, and Josef Neu. *Neonatal and Pediatric Respiratory Care*. St. Louis: Mosby-Year Book, 1993.

Shannon, Margaret T., Billie Ann Wilson, and Carolyn L. Stang. *Health Professional's Drug Guide 2003*. Upper Saddle River, NJ: Prentice Hall, 2003.

Shores, Louis, ed. *Collier's Encyclopedia*. New York: The Crowell-Collier Publishing Company, 1963.

ARTICLES

Cromie, William J. "Cystic Fibrosis Gene Found to Protect Against Typhoid." *The Harvard University Gazette*, July 9, 1998, www.hno.harvard.edu/gazette/1998/07.09/CysticFibrosisG.html.

Denton, Miles. "MRSA in Cystic Fibrosis." Leeds University Teaching Hospitals, UK (May 2001), www.cysticfibrosismedicine.com/htmldocs/CFText/mrsa.htm.

Galdamez, Salvador. "Discovery of the Cystic Fibrosis Gene" (1989), www.quasar.ualberta.ca/edse456/apt/vignettes/cystic.htm.

Jones, Chris. "Goodman's Maggio Dies at 49." *Variety*, August 22, 2000, print.google.com/print/doc?articleid=wTMhy96ukF3.

Littlewood, Jim. "The Historical Development of Nutritional and Dietetic Management of Cystic Fibrosis" (April 2002), www.sustainit.com/cfmain/open/topics/CFText/historydiet.html.

Moran, Antoinette. "Cystic-Fibrosis-related Diabetes." *CF-Related Diabetes* (October 1996), www.cfservicepharmacy .com/homeline_newsletter/archive.index.cfm?articleid=54.

Neergard, Laura. "Spice Substance May Fight Cystic Fibrosis." Associated Press, Washington, DC, April 22, 2004.

Sugg, Diana K. "The Famous Dead Yield Only Murky Diagnosis." *The Sun*, November 17, 2002, www.pulitzer.org/year/2003/beat-reporting/works/sugg6.html.

Whitford, Ben. "An Unexpected Reprieve." *Newsweek*, September 12, 2005.

WEBSITES

ADC Online. Archives of Diseases in Childhood, adc.bmj journals.com/cgi/content/abstract/archdischild%3B84/2/160.

American Biosystems, classes.kumc.edu/cahe/respcared/cybercas/cysticfibrosis/tracpurp.html.

Arizona Respiratory Center, www.resp-sci.arizona.edu/patient-info/child/cystic-fibrosis-k.html.

The Boomer Esiason Foundation, www.esiason.org.

Canadian Cystic Fibrosis Foundation, www.cysticfibrosis.ca/page.asp?id=82.

———. Celine Dion Talks to You, celinedion.t2u.free.fr/celinedion/index.php?lamg=en&page=fk.

CF Info. Information on Selected Aspects of Cystic Fibrosis, www.marketmed.org/cf/cfinfo.htm#polyps.

Cincinnati Children's Hospital Medical Center, www .cincinattichildrens.org/health/info/chest/diagnose/cf-diagnosis.htm.

Cystic Fibrosis Foundation, cff.org.

Cystic Fibrosis Trust, www.cftrust.org.uk/meeting_point/
faqs_adults.htm.

Cystic-L Handbook, www.cystic-L.com/handbook/html/
physical_therapy.htm#Autogenic.

DiabetoValens. Diabetes Matters. "Cystic Fibrosis Related
Diabetes Mellitus," www.mydiabetovalens.com/infocus/
cystic.asp.

Discovery Health. Diseases and Conditions: PICC Line,
www.discovery.com.

Earthlink. Search on Cystic Fibrosis,
search.earthlink.net/search?q=cystic+fibrosis.

History of CF, www3.nbnet.nb.ca/normap/cfhistpry.htm.

Kids Health for Parents, websrv02.kidshealth.org/parent/
medical/digestive/cf.html.

Lucile Packard Children's Hospital at Stanford. Respiratory
Disorders: Cystic Fibrosis and the Respiratory System.
"How Does Cystic Fibrosis Affect the Respiratory System?"
www.lpch.org/diseaseHEalthInfo/HealthLibrary/respire/
cfrespir.html.

Medfacts, "Cystic Fibrosis and Burkholderia Cepacia: B.
Cepacia," www.njc.org/medfacts/cystic.html.

Medicine.net, www.medicinenet.com/dornase_alpha/
article.htm.

NIDDK: Cystic Fibrosis Research Directions,
www.niddk.nih.gov/health/endo/pubs/cystic/cystic.htm.

Norma Kennedy Plourde's Cystic Fibrosis website, personal
.nbnet.nb.ca/normap/CF.htm.

Sweat Testing, www.pediatrics.wisc.edu/patientcare/cf/
sweat.html.

Wijenaike, Nishan, consultant diabetologist. West Suffolk
Diabetes Service (November 2003),
www.diabetesSuffolk.com/Complications/Cystic%20
fibrosis.asp.

WKSU, www.wksu.org/classical/articles/what_killed
_chopin.html.

Yahoo. Search on Celine Dion,
search.yahoo.com/search?x=wrt&p=celebrities+associated
+cystic+fibrosis+&fr=fp-pull-web-t&n=20&fl=0.

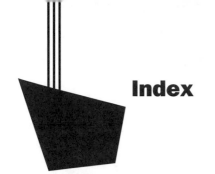

Index

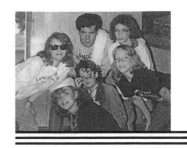

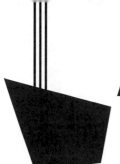

About the Author

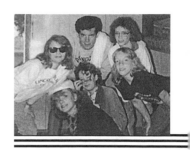

Melanie Ann Apel spent a week at cystic fibrosis overnight camp in 1986. That week changed her life forever. She attended Bradley University and graduated magna cum laude with a bachelor of arts degree in theatre arts. Wanting to dedicate more of her time to children who have CF, Melanie went on to earn a subsequent bachelor's degree in respiratory care from National-Louis University. She worked as a pediatric respiratory therapist at Children's Memorial Hospital in Chicago for six years. Melanie began writing about CF in 1995, launching a freelance writing career. In addition to having written more than forty nonfiction books for children and young adults, Melanie also compiled and wrote the popular pictorial history *Lincoln Park: Chicago*.

Melanie is co-owner and coordinating director of an innovative art studio for children in Chicago called The Paintbrush. In addition, she is frequently found at her computer writing the newsletter for her neighborhood association, for which she sits on the board of directors; organizing her children's playgroups; planning parties and activities for her children; or escorting them to French class, preschool, and other fun kid activities. Of all her accomplishments, though, Melanie is most proud of the two extraordinary little boys who call her "Mommy." Melanie and her little boys live in Chicago. You can reach Melanie at kidlet31@yahoo.com.

03 07